How to Get Enough Nutrition

Norris Hoffman

Table of Contents

Chapter 1

Introduction to Nutrition

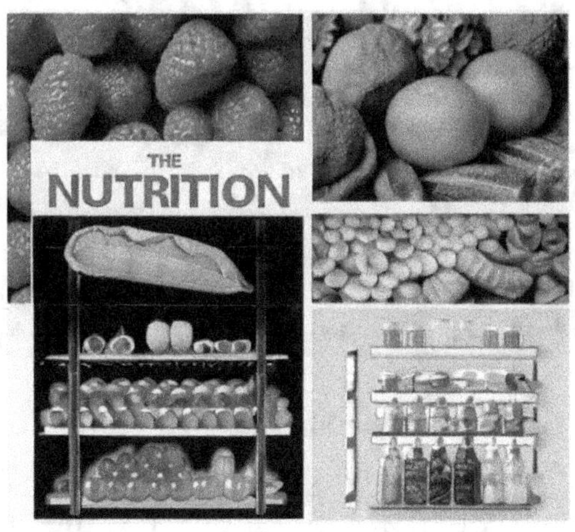

1.1 The Importance of Nutrition for Overall Health and Well-being Legitimate sustenance is fundamental for keeping up with in general wellbeing and prosperity. It provides the body with the necessary nutrients, vitamins, and minerals it needs to function optimally. Good nutrition not only helps in preventing diseases but also plays a crucial role in promoting growth, development, and   longevity.

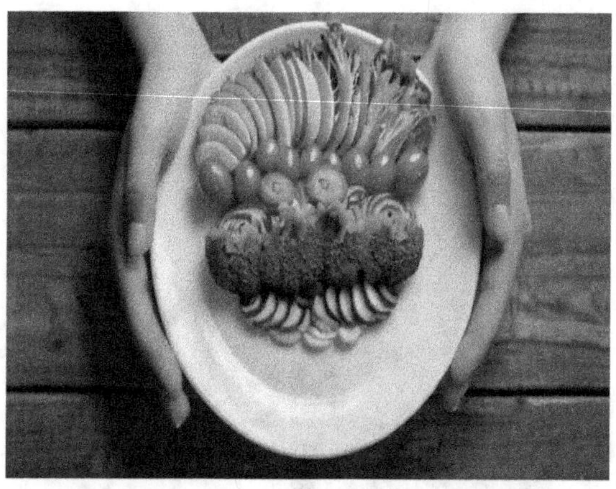

One of the key benefits of nutrition is its impact on energy levels. When we consume a balanced diet that includes all the essential macronutrients and micronutrients, our bodies receive the fuel they need to perform daily activities efficiently. Carbohydrates are the primary source of energy, while proteins help in repairing tissues and building muscles. Fats provide insulation and protect vital organs.

Moreover, proper nutrition supports mental health as well. Studies have shown that certain nutrients can affect brain function and mood regulation. For example, omega-3 fatty acids found in fish have been linked to improved cognitive function and reduced risk of depression. Similarly, B vitamins play a crucial role in neurotransmitter synthesis, which affects mood stability.

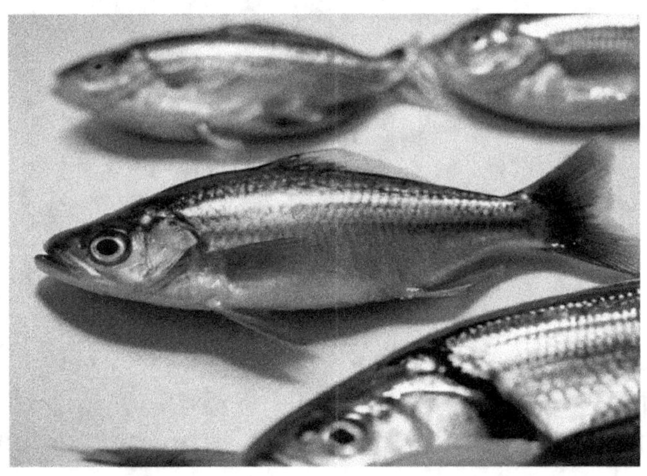

Nutrition also plays a significant role in maintaining a healthy weight. A balanced diet that includes appropriate portions of macronutrients can help prevent obesity and related health issues such as diabetes, heart disease, and joint problems. By understanding portion control and making mindful food choices, individuals can achieve their weight goals while ensuring their bodies receive adequate nutrition.

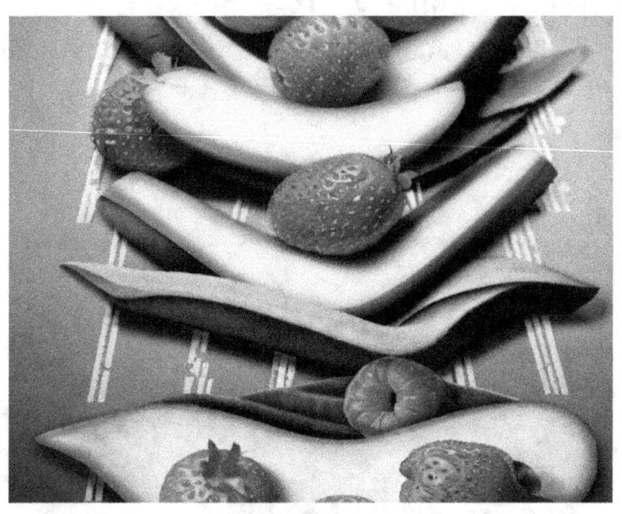

Furthermore, good nutrition is vital for supporting the immune system. A well-nourished body has a stronger defense mechanism against infections and diseases. Nutrients like vitamin C, zinc, selenium, and antioxidants help boost immunity by neutralizing harmful free radicals and supporting cell repair.

To illustrate the importance of nutrition for overall health and well-being, let's consider an example: Sarah is a busy working professional who often relies on fast food or processed meals due to time constraints. As a result, she frequently feels fatigued and lacks the energy to perform daily tasks. Sarah decides to make a change and starts incorporating more whole foods into her diet, including fruits, vegetables, lean proteins, and whole grains. Within a few weeks, she notices a significant improvement in her energy levels and overall well-being. She feels more alert, focused, and motivated throughout the day.

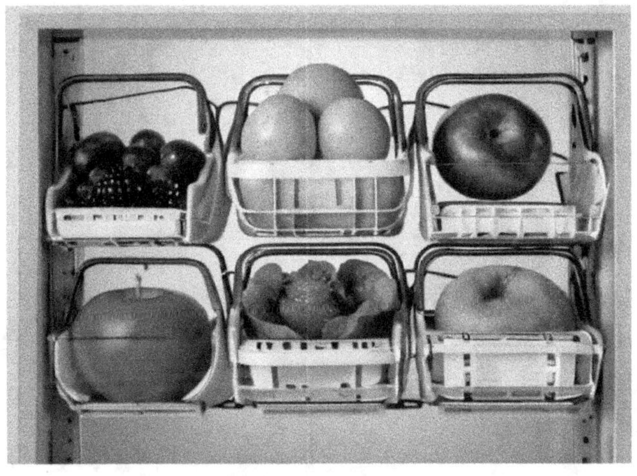

1.2 Understanding Macronutrients and Micronutrients

Macronutrients and micronutrients are essential components of a balanced diet that provide the body with the necessary nutrients for optimal functioning.

Macronutrients include carbohydrates, proteins, and fats. Carbohydrates are the body's primary source of energy and can be found in foods such as grains, fruits, vegetables, and legumes. Proteins are crucial for building and repairing tissues, supporting immune function, and producing enzymes and hormones. Good sources of protein include meat, fish, dairy products, legumes, nuts, and seeds. Fats are essential for insulation, protecting organs, absorbing vitamins A,D,E,K., and providing energy during prolonged exercise or fasting periods. Healthy sources of fats include avocados,nuts,oils,fish etc.

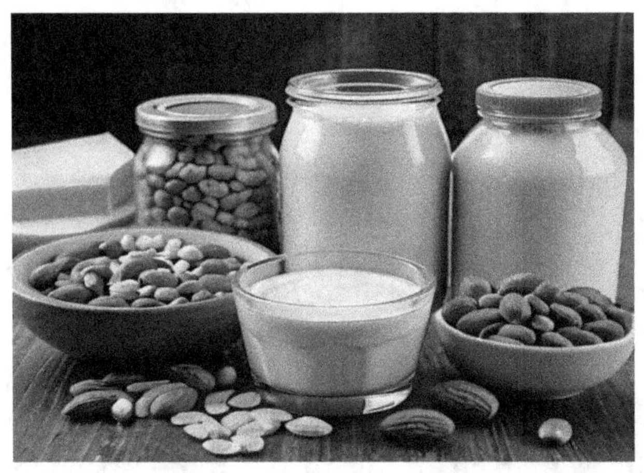

Micronutrients refer to vitamins and minerals that are required in smaller quantities but play vital roles in various bodily functions. Vitamins help regulate metabolism processes such as converting food into energy or maintaining healthy skin cells. Minerals like calcium support bone health while iron is necessary for oxygen transport in the blood.

Understanding macronutrients' role helps individuals make informed choices about their diet composition based on their specific goals or dietary restrictions. For example,a person looking to build muscle may increase their protein intake while someone aiming to lose weight might focus on portion control of carbohydrates.

Similarly,micronutrient knowledge allows individuals to identify potential deficiencies or imbalances in their diet.For instance,a vegetarian who avoids animal products may need to pay extra attention to sources of vitamin B12 or iron.

To further illustrate the importance of macronutrients and micronutrients, let's consider an example: John is a fitness enthusiast who wants to improve his athletic performance. He realizes that he needs to consume an adequate amount of carbohydrates to fuel his workouts and proteins for muscle repair and growth. By incorporating complex carbohydrates like whole grains and lean proteins such as chicken breast into his diet, John notices a significant improvement in his stamina and recovery time.

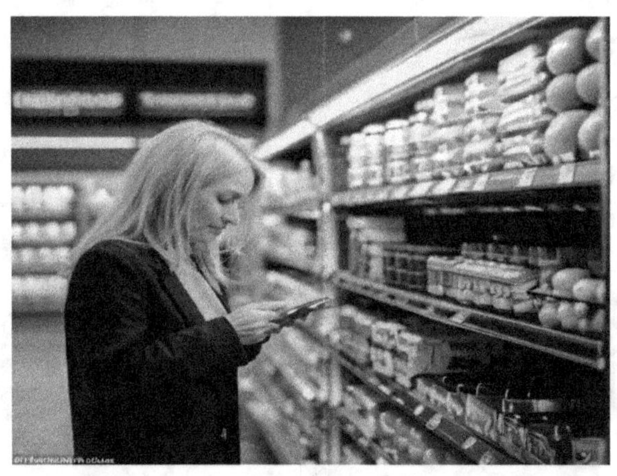

1.3 The Role of Nutrition in Disease Prevention

Nutrition plays a crucial role in disease prevention by providing the body with the necessary tools to fight off infections, maintain healthy bodily functions, and reduce the risk of chronic diseases.

A well-balanced diet rich in fruits, vegetables, whole grains, lean proteins, and healthy fats can help prevent various diseases such as heart disease, diabetes, obesity, certain types of cancer, and osteoporosis. For example,a diet high in fiber from fruits and vegetables can lower the risk of developing heart disease by reducing cholesterol levels. Similarly,a diet low in saturated fats can help prevent obesity and related health issues.

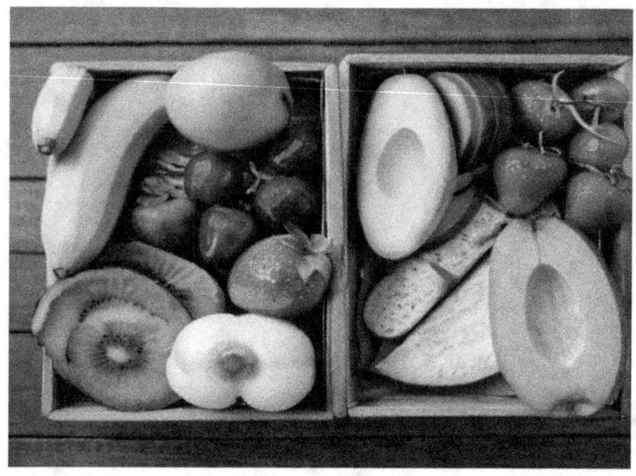

Moreover,nutrition also influences our gut health which has been linked to various diseases including autoimmune disorders like Crohn's disease or ulcerative colitis. A healthy gut microbiome is essential for proper digestion and absorption of nutrients while also supporting immune function.

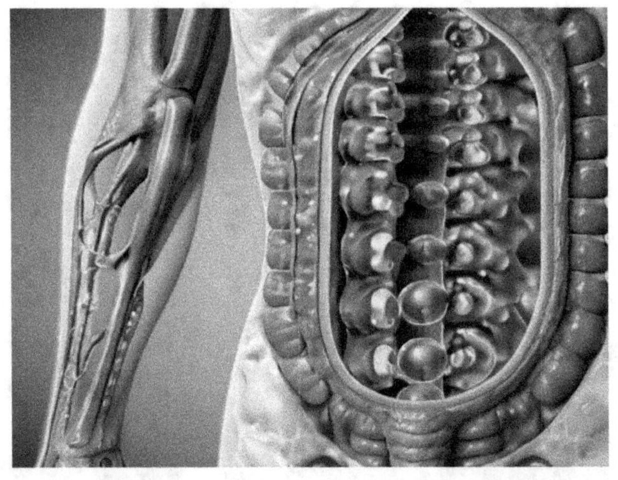

Additionally,some specific nutrients have been found to have protective effects against certain diseases.For instance,vitamin D has been associated with a reduced risk of multiple sclerosis while antioxidants like vitamin C,E or beta-carotene may help protect against certain cancers.

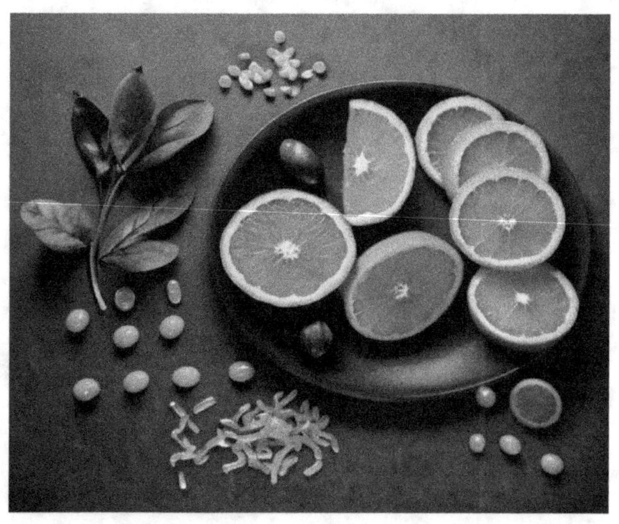

To highlight the role of nutrition in disease prevention, let's consider an example: Lisa has a family history of heart disease,and she wants to take proactive steps to reduce her risk.She starts following a heart-healthy diet that includes plenty of fruits,vegetables,fish,and whole grains while limiting her intake of saturated fats and processed foods. Over time,Lisa's cholesterol levels improve,and she feels more confident about her heart health.

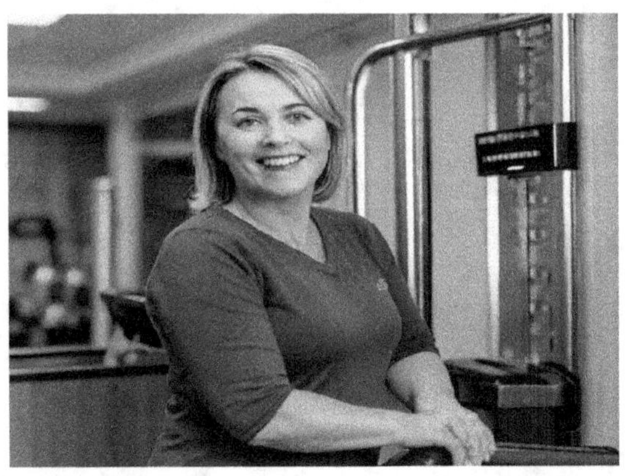

In conclusion, nutrition is vital for overall health and well-being as it provides the body with essential nutrients, supports energy levels, mental health, weight management, and immune function. Understanding macronutrients and micronutrients helps individuals make informed choices about their diet composition based on their goals or dietary restrictions. Furthermore, nutrition plays a significant role in disease prevention by reducing the risk of chronic diseases and supporting optimal bodily functions. By prioritizing proper nutrition, individuals can enhance their quality of life and promote long-term health.

Chapter 2

Expert Insights on Nutrition

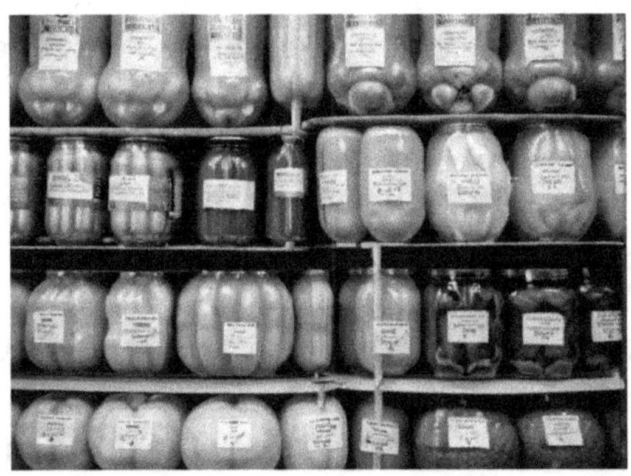

2.1 Gathering Information from Experts in the Field of Nutrition

When it comes to writing a book on nutrition, gathering information from experts in the field is crucial. These experts have dedicated their lives to studying and understanding the complexities of nutrition, and their insights can provide valuable guidance for creating an informative and accurate book.

One effective way to gather information from experts is through interviews or consultations. By directly speaking with experts, authors can gain firsthand knowledge and insights that may not be readily available in existing research or literature. These interviews can delve into specific topics or address any questions or concerns that arise during the writing process.

Another approach is to attend conferences or seminars where experts in nutrition are presenting their research findings. These events provide an opportunity to learn about the latest advancements and trends in the field. Additionally, networking with other attendees can lead to connections with experts who may be willing to contribute their expertise to the book.

Incorporating case studies or real-world examples can also enhance the credibility and practicality of the book. By showcasing individuals who have successfully implemented nutritional strategies into their lives, readers can see firsthand how proper nutrition can positively impact health and well-being.

Furthermore, it is important to consider diverse perspectives when gathering information from experts. Nutrition is a complex field with various schools of thought and differing opinions on certain topics. By seeking out a range of expert opinions, authors can present a more comprehensive view of nutrition, allowing readers to make informed decisions based on different perspectives.

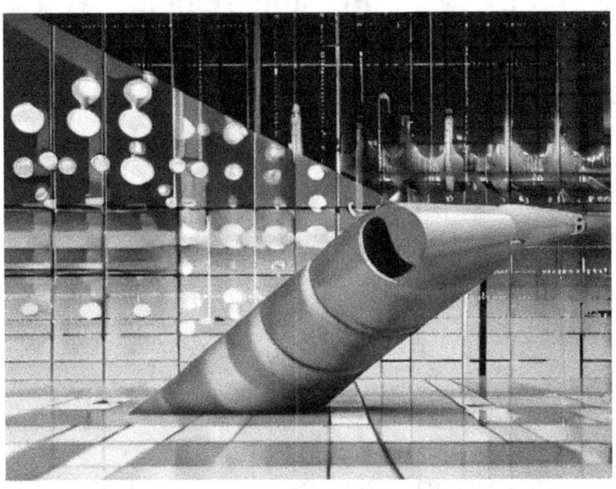

Overall, gathering information from experts in the field of nutrition involves conducting interviews or consultations, attending conferences or seminars, incorporating case studies or real-world examples, and considering diverse perspectives. By utilizing these approaches, authors can ensure that their book provides accurate and valuable insights into achieving optimal nutrition.

2.2 Determining Topics to Address in the Book

Determining which topics to address in a book on nutrition requires careful consideration of the target audience's needs and interests, as well as an understanding of current trends and research in the field. By addressing relevant and timely topics, authors can provide readers with valuable information that is both informative and practical.

One approach to determining topics is to conduct a thorough analysis of existing books on nutrition. By studying these books, authors can identify common themes and topics that have been extensively covered. This analysis allows authors to identify gaps in the existing literature and focus on areas that have not been adequately addressed.

Additionally, conducting keyword research can help determine popular topics related to nutrition. By analyzing search engine data or using keyword research tools, authors can identify the most frequently searched terms or phrases related to nutrition. This insight can guide the selection of topics that are highly relevant and in demand among readers.

Another effective approach is to consider emerging trends in the field of nutrition. As new research and discoveries are made, certain topics may gain prominence or become more relevant. For example, with the rise of plant-based diets, addressing the benefits and challenges of adopting such a diet could be a timely topic for inclusion in the book.

Furthermore, it is important to consider the specific needs and interests of the target audience when determining topics. Conducting surveys or focus groups can provide valuable insights into what readers are looking for in a book on nutrition. Understanding their concerns, goals, and preferences will help shape the content to meet their needs effectively.

Lastly, it is essential to strike a balance between covering fundamental concepts and exploring more advanced or specialized topics. Beginners may require basic information on macronutrients, micronutrients, meal planning, and portion control. However, more experienced individuals may be interested in topics such as sports nutrition or nutritional strategies for specific health conditions.

In conclusion, determining topics to address in a book on nutrition involves analyzing existing literature, conducting keyword research, considering emerging trends in the field, understanding the target audience's needs and interests, and striking a balance between fundamental and advanced topics. By utilizing these approaches, authors can ensure that their book covers relevant and valuable information that resonates with readers.

2.3 Effective Approaches for Reaching the Target Audience

Reaching the target audience is crucial for the success of any book on nutrition. To effectively engage readers and ensure that the book's message reaches its intended audience, authors must employ various strategies and approaches tailored to their specific demographic.

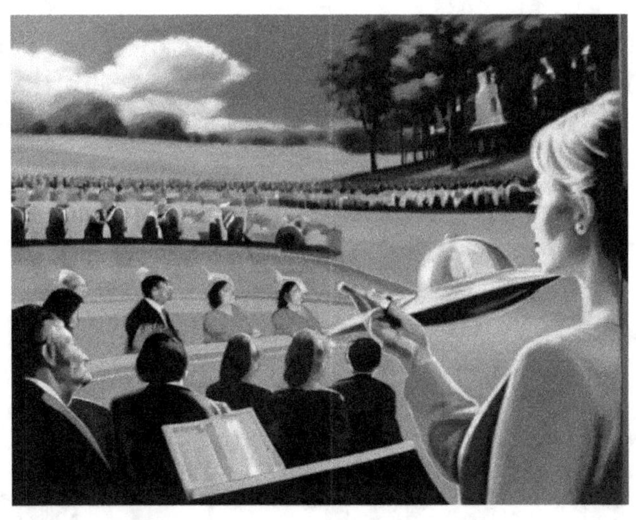

One effective approach is to utilize social media platforms to connect with the target audience. Platforms such as Instagram, Facebook, Twitter, and YouTube provide opportunities to share valuable content, engage in discussions, and build a community around the book's topic. By consistently posting informative and engaging content, authors can attract followers who are interested in nutrition and increase awareness of their book.

Collaborating with influencers or experts in the field of nutrition can also help reach a wider audience. Influencers often have a dedicated following who trust their recommendations and insights. By partnering with influencers or experts, authors can tap into their existing audience base and leverage their credibility to promote the book.

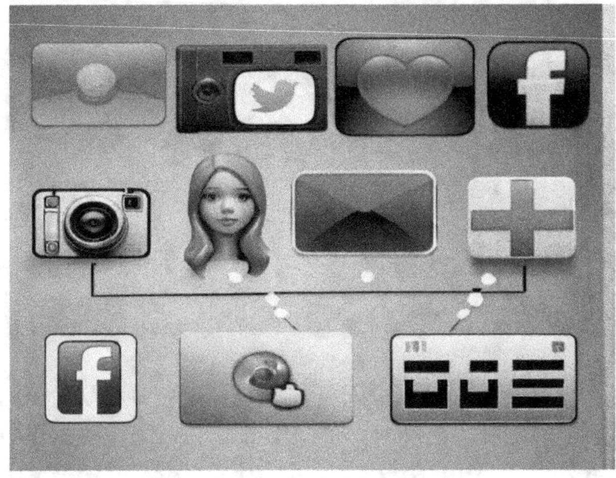

Another effective approach is to offer free resources or samples related to the book's content. This could include downloadable meal plans, recipe guides, or educational videos. By providing valuable resources for free, authors can demonstrate their expertise while also enticing readers to purchase the full book for more comprehensive information.

Utilizing email marketing campaigns can also be an effective way to reach the target audience. By collecting email addresses through website sign-ups or social media promotions, authors can send regular newsletters or updates about the book's release or additional resources. This direct communication allows authors to maintain engagement with readers over time.

Additionally, considering different formats for reaching the target audience can expand the book's reach. For example, creating an audiobook version of the text allows individuals who prefer listening over reading to access the content. Exploring partnerships with podcasters or hosting webinars can also provide opportunities to engage with the target audience in a more interactive and dynamic manner.

Lastly, leveraging traditional media outlets such as newspapers, magazines, or radio shows can help reach a broader audience. By pitching the book's content or offering to contribute articles or interviews, authors can gain exposure to readers who may not be actively seeking nutrition-related information online.

In conclusion, effective approaches for reaching the target audience include utilizing social media platforms, collaborating with influencers or experts, offering free resources or samples, implementing email marketing campaigns, considering different formats for content delivery, and leveraging traditional media outlets. By employing these strategies tailored to the specific demographic of the target audience, authors can effectively promote their book and ensure that it reaches its intended readership.

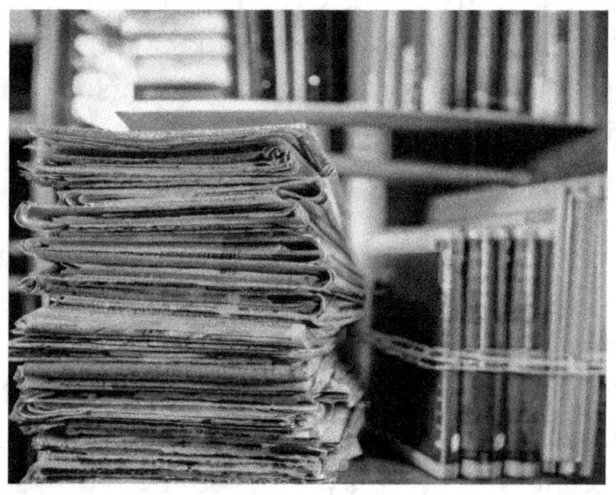

Chapter 3

Getting Started with Proper Nutrition

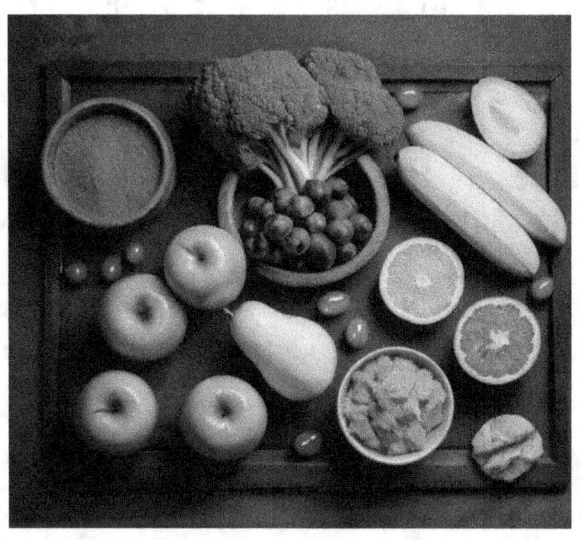

3.1 Assessing Your Current Diet and Nutritional Needs

Assessing your current diet and nutritional needs is an essential first step in achieving optimal nutrition. It allows you to understand where you currently stand in terms of your nutrient intake and identify any deficiencies or imbalances that may exist. By conducting a thorough assessment, you can make informed decisions about the changes you need to make to improve your diet.

One way to assess your current diet is by keeping a food diary for a week. Write down everything you eat and drink, including portion sizes and preparation methods. This will give you a clear picture of your eating habits and help you identify patterns or areas where improvements can be made. For example, you may notice that you consume too many processed foods or that your vegetable intake is lacking.

Another important aspect of assessing your nutritional needs is understanding the specific requirements for different nutrients based on factors such as age, sex, weight, activity level, and any underlying health conditions. Consulting with a registered dietitian or nutritionist can provide valuable insights into your individual nutritional needs. They can analyze your dietary intake, consider any specific health concerns, and provide personalized recommendations tailored to your unique circumstances.

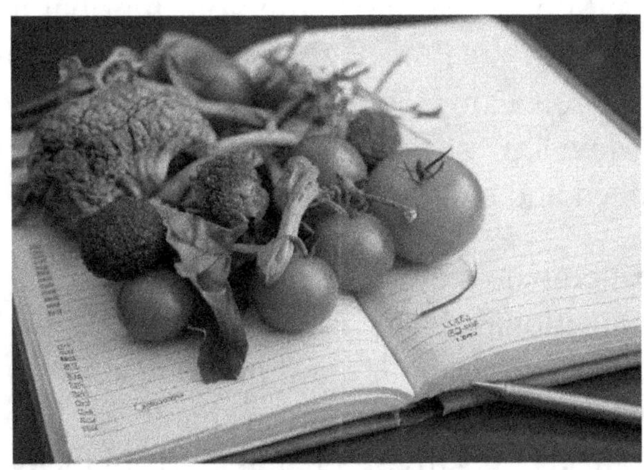

It's also crucial to consider any cultural or personal preferences when assessing your current diet. For example, if you follow a vegetarian or vegan lifestyle, it's important to ensure that you are meeting all the necessary nutrient requirements through plant-based sources. Similarly, if you have certain food allergies or intolerances, it's essential to find suitable alternatives that still provide the required nutrients.

In addition to evaluating what you eat, it's equally important to assess how you eat. Factors such as meal timing, portion control, and mindful eating practices play a significant role in achieving optimal nutrition. For instance, if you tend to skip meals or eat irregularly throughout the day, it may be impacting your nutrient intake and overall health. By assessing your eating habits, you can identify areas for improvement and develop strategies to establish a more balanced and consistent eating routine.

Remember that assessing your current diet and nutritional needs is not about judgment or criticism. It's about gaining awareness and understanding of your current habits so that you can make positive changes. Embrace this process as an opportunity for growth and improvement, knowing that small adjustments can lead to significant long-term benefits for your health.

3.2 Setting Goals for Achieving Optimal Nutrition

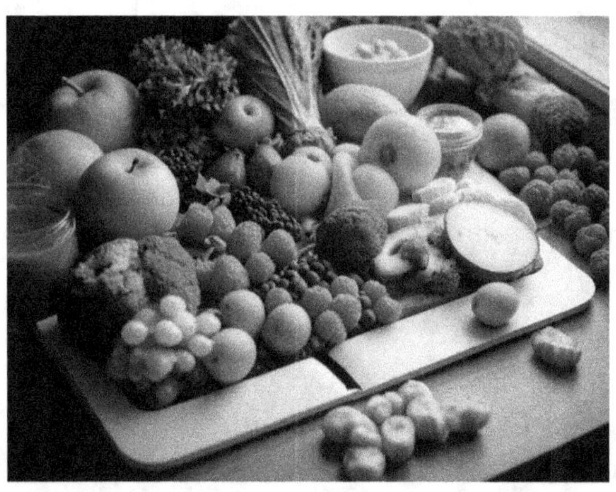

Setting goals is a crucial step in achieving optimal nutrition. Without clear objectives, it can be challenging to stay motivated and track progress towards improving your diet. By setting explicit, quantifiable, reachable, significant, and time-bound (Brilliant) objectives, you can make a guide for progress.

When setting goals for optimal nutrition, it's important to consider both short-term and long-term objectives. Short-term goals provide immediate targets that are easier to achieve, while long-term goals help guide your overall journey towards better nutrition. For example, a short-term goal could be to increase your daily vegetable intake by one serving within the next week, while a long-term goal could be to maintain a balanced diet consistently over the next six months.

To ensure that your goals are realistic and attainable, it's essential to take into account your current lifestyle, commitments, and resources. For instance, if you have a busy schedule with limited time for meal preparation, setting a goal of cooking all meals from scratch may not be feasible initially. Instead, you could start by incorporating one homemade meal per day and gradually increase as you become more comfortable with the process.

It's also important to make your goals specific rather than vague or general. Instead of saying "I want to eat healthier," specify what that means for you personally. For example, you could set a goal of reducing added sugar intake by swapping sugary drinks with infused water or herbal tea. This specificity helps you focus on actionable steps and measure progress more effectively.

In addition to setting goals related to specific nutrients or food groups, it's beneficial to consider behavioral goals that support healthy eating habits. For example, you could set a goal of practicing mindful eating by slowing down during meals, savoring each bite, and paying attention to hunger and fullness cues. These behavioral goals can have a significant impact on your overall relationship with food and contribute to long-term success in achieving optimal nutrition.

Remember that setting goals is not about perfection or strict adherence to a rigid plan. It's about creating a framework that guides your decision-making and provides direction towards better nutrition. Be flexible and open to adjusting your goals as needed, recognizing that progress is more important than perfection.

3.3 Overcoming Challenges and Barriers to Proper Nutrition

Proper nutrition can sometimes be challenging due to various barriers that may exist in our daily lives. However, with the right strategies and mindset, these challenges can be overcome, allowing us to achieve optimal nutrition.

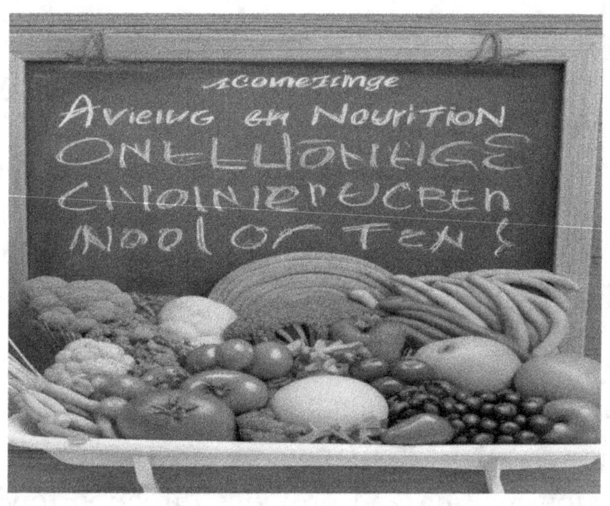

One common barrier to proper nutrition is time constraints. Many people lead busy lives with packed schedules, making it difficult to prioritize meal planning, grocery shopping, and cooking nutritious meals. To overcome this challenge, it's essential to prioritize and allocate time specifically for these activities. Consider meal prepping on weekends or utilizing time-saving techniques such as batch cooking or using slow cookers. By planning ahead and being organized, you can ensure that nutritious meals are readily available even during hectic times.

Another challenge is the availability of unhealthy food options in our environment.

Processed foods high in sugar, salt, and unhealthy fats are often more accessible and affordable than fresh produce or whole foods. To overcome this barrier, it's important to make conscious choices when grocery shopping and opt for nutrient-dense foods whenever possible. Additionally, finding healthier alternatives or preparing homemade versions of favorite dishes can help navigate through the abundance of unhealthy options.

Lack of knowledge or misinformation about nutrition can also pose a significant barrier. With such a lot of clashing data accessible, isolating truth from fiction can be challenging. To overcome this challenge, it's crucial to seek reliable sources of information such as registered dietitians, reputable websites, or evidence-based books and articles. Educating yourself about the basics of nutrition and understanding the science behind it can empower you to make informed choices and navigate through the sea of misinformation.

Another common barrier is emotional eating or using food as a coping mechanism for stress, boredom, or other emotions. Overcoming emotional eating requires developing alternative coping strategies and addressing the underlying emotional triggers. This may involve seeking support from a therapist or counselor who specializes in emotional eating or practicing stress management techniques such as meditation, exercise, or engaging in hobbies that bring joy and fulfillment.

Lastly, social pressures and cultural norms can also present challenges to proper nutrition. For example, attending social gatherings where unhealthy foods are abundant can make it difficult to stick to your nutritional goals. In these situations, it's important to communicate your dietary preferences or restrictions with friends and family members in advance. Additionally, bringing a healthy dish to share at gatherings ensures that you have an option that aligns with your goals.

In conclusion, overcoming challenges and barriers to proper nutrition requires awareness, planning, and perseverance. By identifying specific obstacles that may hinder your progress and implementing strategies tailored to your circumstances, you can navigate through these challenges successfully. Remember that change takes time and effort but is well worth it for the long-term benefits to your health and well-being.

Chapter 4

Understanding Macronutrients

4.1 Carbohydrates: The Body's Main Source of Energy

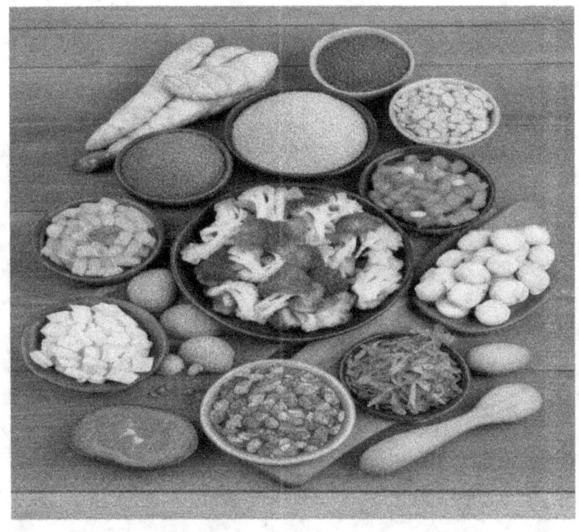

Carbohydrates are often misunderstood and unfairly demonized in popular diets. However, they are actually the body's main source of energy and play a crucial role in maintaining overall health and well-being. Carbohydrates are found in a variety of foods such as grains, fruits, vegetables, and dairy products.

One important aspect to understand about carbohydrates is their classification into straightforward and complex sugars. Straightforward starches, otherwise called sugars, are immediately processed and give a quick explosion of energy. Examples include table sugar, honey, and fruit juices. Then again, complex starches consist of longer chains of sugar molecules that take longer to break down. These include whole grains, legumes, and starchy vegetables.

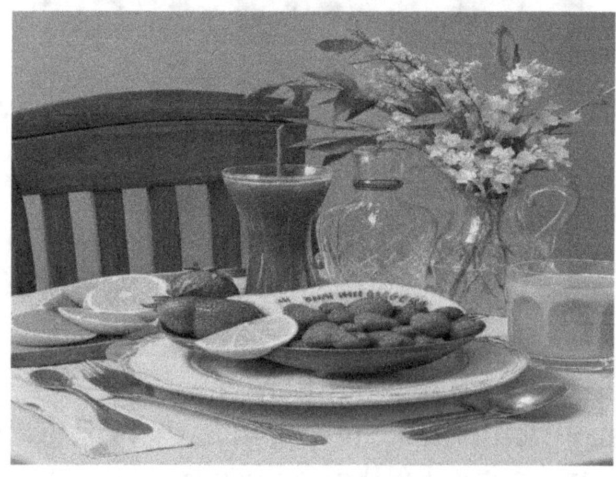

It is essential to consume a balanced mix of both simple and complex carbohydrates to ensure sustained energy levels throughout the day. For example, starting your day with a bowl of oatmeal topped with fresh berries provides a combination of complex carbohydrates for long-lasting energy along with simple carbohydrates from the natural sugars in the fruit.

Furthermore, it is important to consider the glycemic index (GI) when choosing carbohydrate-rich foods.The GI estimates how rapidly a specific food raises glucose levels. Foods with a high GI cause a rapid spike in blood sugar levels followed by a crash in energy levels shortly after consumption. On the other hand, low GI foods provide more stable energy levels over an extended period.

For instance, opting for whole grain bread instead of white bread can help maintain steady blood sugar levels due to its lower GI value. This can prevent sudden drops in energy and reduce cravings for unhealthy snacks between meals.

In addition to providing energy, carbohydrates also contribute to brain function. The cerebrum depends intensely on glucose as its essential fuel source. When carbohydrate intake is inadequate or restricted for prolonged periods, cognitive function may be impaired, leading to difficulties in concentration and memory.It is essential to take note of that not all carbs are made equivalent. Processed and refined carbohydrates, such as white bread, sugary cereals, and pastries, should be limited as they lack essential nutrients and can contribute to weight gain and chronic diseases like diabetes. Instead, focus on consuming whole foods that are rich in fiber, vitamins, and minerals.

4.2 Proteins: Building Blocks for Growth and Repair

Proteins are often referred to as the building blocks of life because they play a crucial role in the growth, repair, and maintenance of tissues in the body. They are made up of amino acids, which are linked together in various combinations to form different proteins.

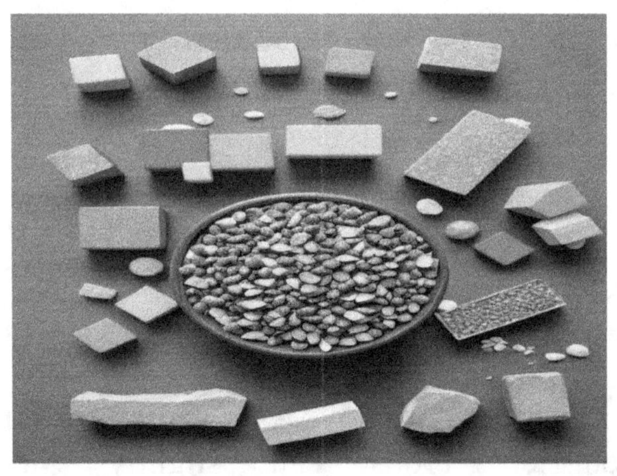

There are two primary kinds of dietary protein: complete proteins and deficient proteins. Complete proteins contain each of the nine fundamental amino acids that the body can't deliver all alone. Animal-based sources such as meat, fish, eggs, and dairy products are considered complete proteins. On the other hand, plant-based sources like legumes, grains, nuts, and seeds are generally incomplete proteins but can be combined to provide all essential amino acids.

Protein intake is particularly important for individuals who engage in regular physical activity or strength training. During exercise or resistance training, muscle fibers undergo microscopic damage that needs to be repaired for muscle growth and recovery. Adequate protein consumption provides the necessary amino acids for this repair process.

Moreover, protein has a higher thermic effect compared to carbohydrates or fats. This means that it requires more energy for digestion and absorption by the body. As a result, consuming protein-rich foods can slightly increase metabolism compared to other macronutrients.

It is worth noting that excessive protein intake does not necessarily equate to better results. The body has a limit on how much protein it can effectively utilize for muscle synthesis and repair. Consuming excessive amounts of protein beyond this limit may strain the kidneys and liver, leading to potential health issues.

To optimize protein intake, it is recommended to distribute protein consumption evenly throughout the day. This ensures a steady supply of amino acids for muscle repair and growth. Including a source of protein in each meal and snack can help achieve this balance. For example, adding Greek yogurt or cottage cheese to a fruit salad provides a combination of carbohydrates and protein for sustained energy and muscle recovery.

4.3 Fats: Essential for Energy Storage and Hormone Production

Fats often have a negative reputation due to their association with weight gain and cardiovascular diseases. However, fats are an essential macronutrient that plays several vital roles in the body. They provide energy, support cell growth, protect organs, insulate the body, and aid in hormone production.

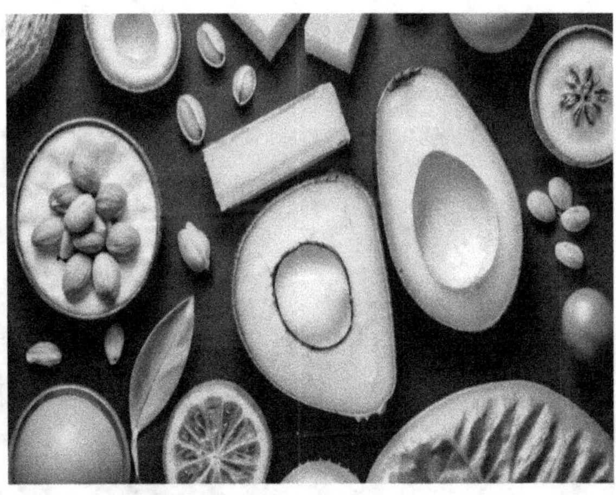

There are different types of dietary fats: saturated fats, unsaturated fats (including monounsaturated and polyunsaturated fats), and trans fats. Saturated fats are commonly found in animal products such as meat, dairy products, and tropical oils like coconut oil. Unsaturated fats are mainly found in plant-based sources such as avocados, nuts, seeds, olive oil, and fatty fish like salmon.

It is important to focus on consuming healthy sources of fat while limiting unhealthy ones. Saturated fats should be consumed in moderation as excessive intake has been linked to an increased risk of heart disease. On the other hand, unsaturated fats have been associated with various health benefits including improved heart health when consumed in appropriate amounts.

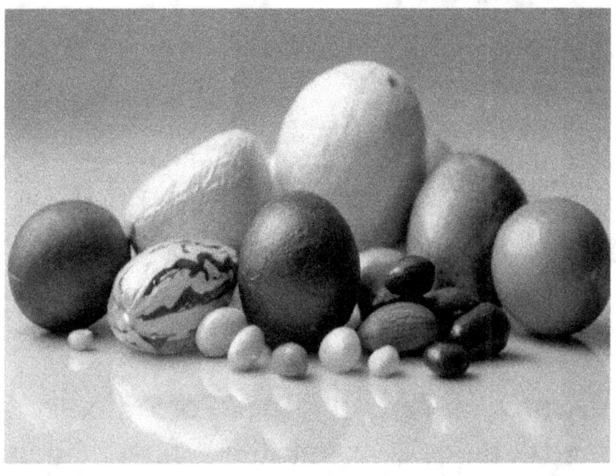

Omega-3 fatty acids are a type of polyunsaturated fat that has gained significant attention due to its numerous health benefits. These fatty acids are primarily found in fatty fish like salmon, mackerel, sardines, as well as flaxseeds and walnuts. Omega-3s have been shown to reduce inflammation in the body, improve brain function, support heart health by reducing triglyceride levels, and even alleviate symptoms of depression.

Incorporating healthy fats into the diet can be as simple as drizzling olive oil over a salad or adding avocado slices to a sandwich. These small changes not only enhance the flavor and texture of meals but also provide essential nutrients and promote satiety.

It is important to note that while fats are an essential part of a balanced diet, they are also calorie-dense. Consuming excessive amounts of fat can lead to weight gain if not balanced with appropriate physical activity and overall calorie intake. Control is key with regards to fat utilization.

In conclusion, carbohydrates, proteins, and fats are all essential macronutrients that play unique roles in the body. Carbohydrates provide energy, proteins support growth and repair, and fats contribute to energy storage and hormone production. By understanding the importance of each macronutrient and making informed choices about their sources and quantities, individuals can optimize their nutrition for better health and well-being.

Chapter 5

Understanding Micronutrients

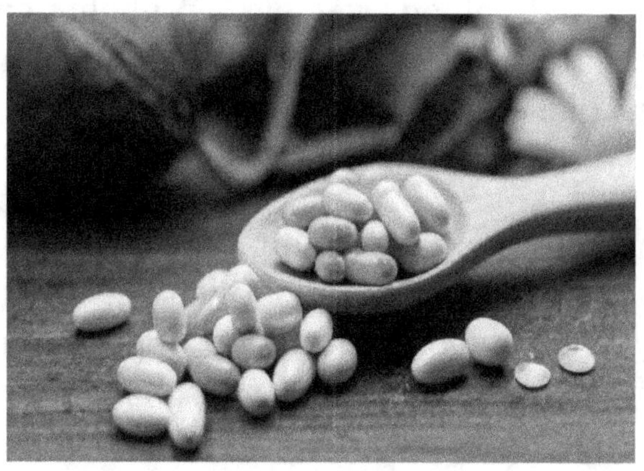

5.1 Vitamins: Essential for Various Body Functions

Nutrients are natural mixtures that are fundamental for different body capabilities. They assume a vital part in keeping up with generally speaking wellbeing and prosperity. While vitamins are required in small amounts, their absence or deficiency can lead to serious health problems.

One of the most well-known vitamins is vitamin C, which is known for its immune-boosting properties. It helps protect the body against infections and promotes the production of collagen, a protein that supports healthy skin, bones, and blood vessels. Without enough vitamin C, individuals may experience side effects like exhaustion, debilitated invulnerable framework, and slow twisted recuperating.

Another important vitamin is vitamin D, often referred to as the "sunshine vitamin." It plays a vital role in bone health by aiding in the absorption of calcium and phosphorus from the diet. Vitamin D deficiency can lead to conditions like rickets in children and osteoporosis in adults. While sunlight is a natural source of vitamin D, it can also be obtained through certain foods or supplements.

Vitamin A is essential for maintaining good vision and promoting healthy skin. It is found in orange-colored fruits and vegetables like carrots and sweet potatoes. Deficiency of vitamin A can lead to night blindness and dry skin.

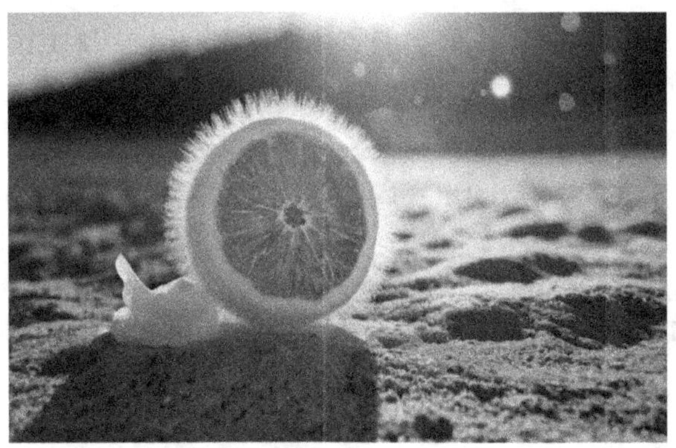

B vitamins are a group of vitamins that play a crucial role in energy production, brain function, and cell metabolism. They incorporate thiamine (B1), riboflavin (B2), niacin (B3), pantothenic corrosive (B5), pyridoxine (B6), biotin (B7), folate (B9), and cobalamin (B12). Each B side effects like exhaustion, debilitated invulnerable framework, and slow twisted recuperating.

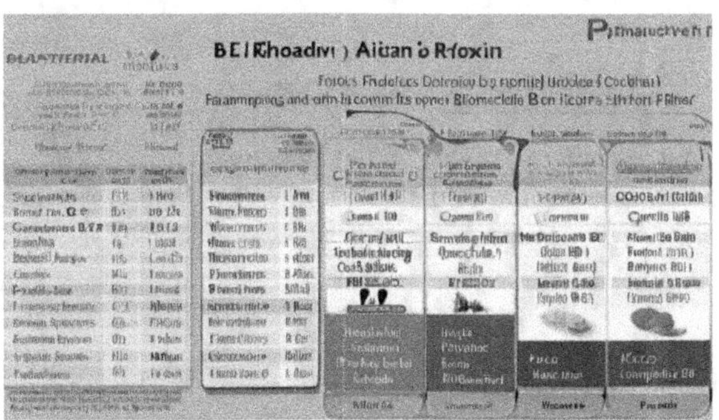

It's important to note that while vitamins are necessary for our bodies to function properly, excessive intake can also be harmful. For example, excessive intake of vitamin A can lead to toxicity and cause symptoms such as nausea, dizziness, and even hair loss. Therefore, it is crucial to maintain a balanced intake of vitamins through a varied and nutritious diet.

5.2 Minerals: Supporting Bone Health, Immune System, and More

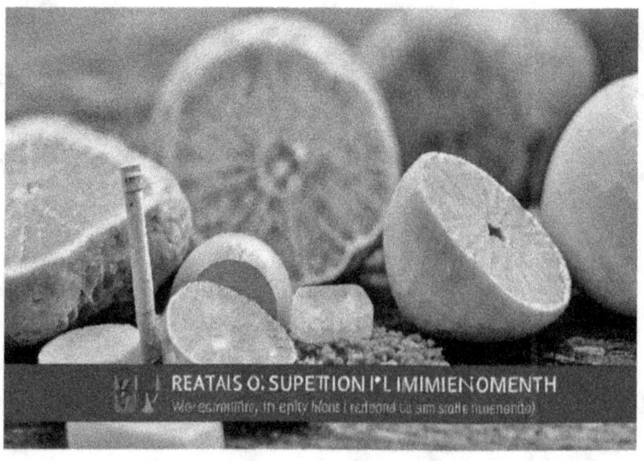

Minerals are inorganic substances that are fundamental for different physical processes. They play a vital role in supporting bone health, maintaining fluid balance, and ensuring proper nerve function.

Calcium is one of the most well-known minerals when it comes to bone health. It is fundamental for the turn of events and upkeep of solid bones and teeth. Calcium deficiency can lead to conditions like osteoporosis, where bones become weak and brittle.Great wellsprings of calcium incorporate dairy items, verdant green vegetables, and sustained food varieties.

Iron is another important mineral that plays a crucial role in carrying oxygen throughout the body. It is an essential component of hemoglobin, the protein responsible for transporting oxygen in red blood cells. Iron deficiency can lead to anemia, characterized by fatigue, weakness, and decreased immune function. Foods rich in iron include lean meats, beans, spinach, and fortified cereals.

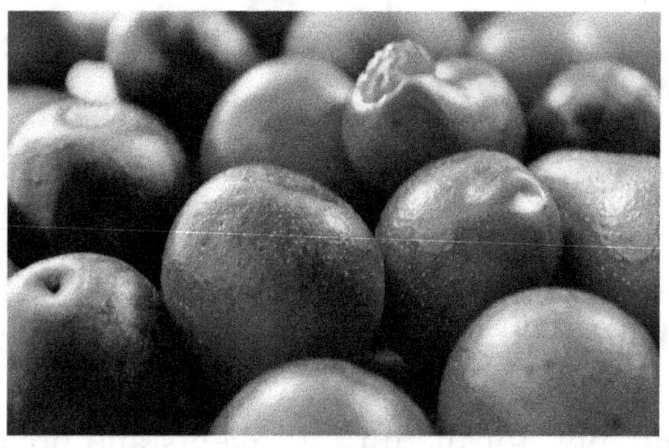

Zinc is a mineral that supports immune function and helps with wound healing. It also plays a role in cell division and growth. Zinc deficiency can impair immune function and delay wound healing. Great wellsprings of zinc incorporate clams, meat, poultry, nuts, and seeds.Magnesium is related with in excess of 300 biochemical reactions in the body. It assumes a critical part in energy creation, muscle capability, and keeping up with typical circulatory strain levels. Lack of magnesium can prompt side effects, for example, muscle issues, weakness, and sporadic heartbeat. Good sources of magnesium include whole grains, nuts/seeds (especially almonds), legumes (such as black beans), dark chocolate/cocoa powder.

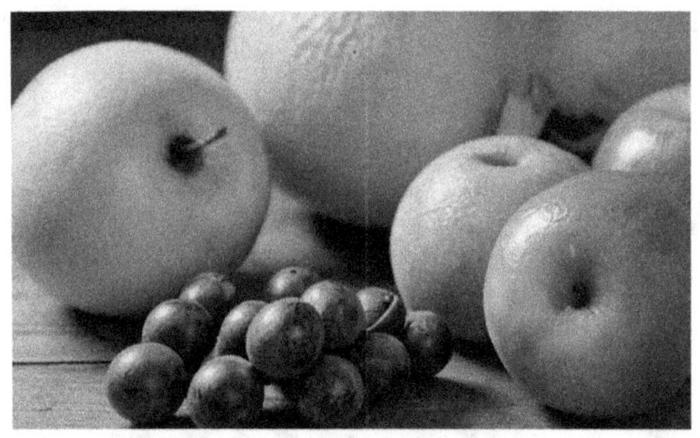

Selenium is a fundamental mineral that goes about as a cancer prevention agent, safeguarding cells from harm brought about by free extremists. It also plays a role in thyroid function and immune system health. Selenium deficiency can lead to weakened immune function and increased risk of certain diseases. Good sources of selenium include Brazil nuts, seafood, meat, and whole grains.

It's important to note that minerals work synergistically with vitamins and other nutrients in the body. Therefore, it is crucial to maintain a balanced intake of minerals through a varied diet that includes a wide range of nutrient-dense foods.

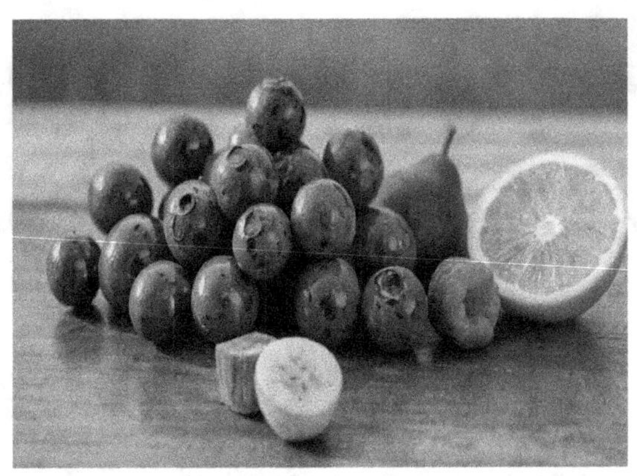

5.3 Antioxidants: Protecting Cells from Damage

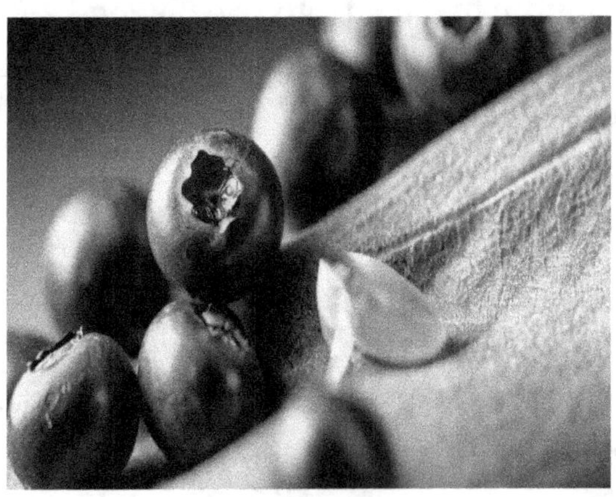

Cancer prevention agents are intensified to assist with shielding cells from harm brought about by free extremists. Free radicals are unstable molecules that can cause oxidative stress, leading to cell damage and potentially contributing to the development of chronic diseases such as heart disease, cancer, and neurodegenerative disorders.

One well-known antioxidant is vitamin C, which we discussed earlier in the section on vitamins. Vitamin C helps neutralize free radicals and regenerate other antioxidants in the body. It is found in citrus natural products, berries, kiwi, peppers, and verdant green vegetables.

Vitamin E is another powerful antioxidant that protects cell membranes from oxidative damage. It cooperates with L-ascorbic acid to improve its cancer prevention agent impacts. Good sources of vitamin E include nuts/seeds (especially almonds), vegetable oils (such as sunflower oil), spinach, and broccoli.

Beta-carotene is a precursor to vitamin A and acts as an antioxidant itself. It gives fruits and vegetables their vibrant orange or yellow color. Beta-carotene-rich foods include carrots, sweet potatoes, apricots, mangoes, and spinach.

Selenium is not only an essential mineral but also acts as an antioxidant by helping to regenerate other antioxidants like vitamin C and vitamin E. As mentioned earlier in the section on minerals, good sources of selenium include Brazil nuts, seafood, meat, and whole grains.

In addition to these specific antioxidants found in vitamins and minerals, there are many other compounds with antioxidant properties found in plant-based foods. These include flavonoids, resveratrol, and anthocyanins, which are found in fruits, vegetables, whole grains, and herbs/spices.

Consuming a diet rich in antioxidants can help reduce the risk of chronic diseases and promote overall health. It is important to note that while antioxidant supplements are available, it is generally recommended to obtain antioxidants through a varied diet rather than relying solely on supplements. This is because whole foods contain a wide range of beneficial compounds that work together synergistically to provide optimal health benefits.

In conclusion, vitamins, minerals, and antioxidants play crucial roles in maintaining overall health and well-being. They support various body functions such as immune function, bone health, energy production, and cell protection. By incorporating a variety of nutrient-dense foods into our diets, we can ensure an adequate intake of these micronutrients and reap the benefits they offer for our bodies.

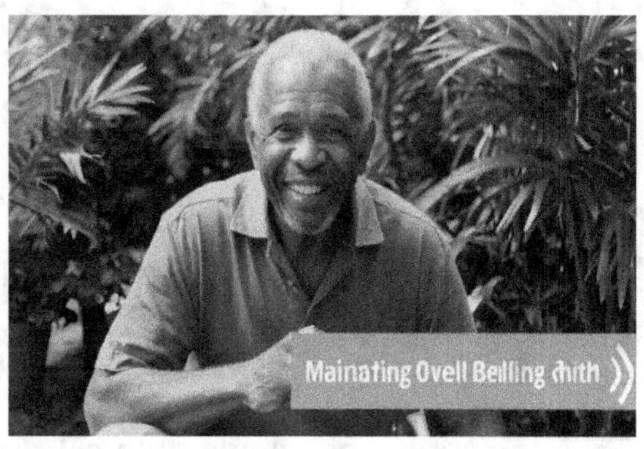

Chapter 6

Meal Planning for Optimal Nutrition

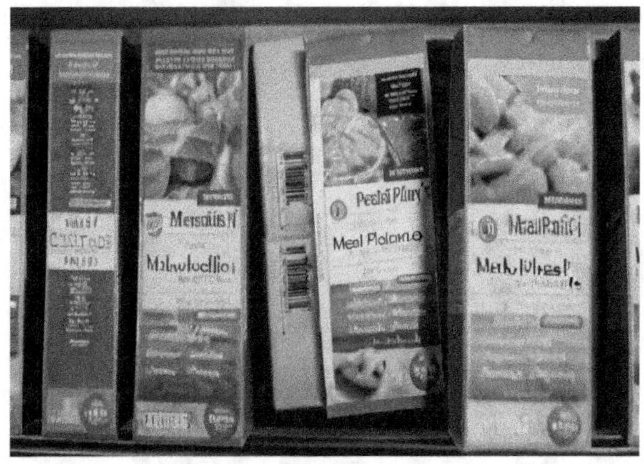

6.1 Creating Balanced Meals with a Variety of Nutrient-rich Foods

Creating balanced meals with a variety of nutrient-rich foods is essential for achieving optimal nutrition. A balanced meal consists of a combination of macronutrients (carbohydrates, proteins, and fats) and micronutrients (vitamins and minerals) that provide the body with the necessary fuel and building blocks for optimal functioning.

When planning your meals, it is important to include a variety of nutrient-rich foods from different food groups. This ensures that you are getting a wide range of essential nutrients that support various bodily functions. For example, incorporating fruits and vegetables into your meals provides vitamins, minerals, and antioxidants that promote overall health and reduce the risk of chronic diseases.

To create balanced meals, consider the following   tips:

- 1.Include a source of lean protein: Protein is crucial for muscle repair and growth, as well as for maintaining healthy skin, hair, and nails. Choose lean sources such as chicken breast, fish, tofu, or legumes to minimize saturated fat intake.
- 2.Incorporate whole grains: Whole grains are rich in fiber, which aids digestion and helps regulate blood sugar

levels. Opt for whole wheat bread, brown rice, quinoa, or oats instead of refined grains like white bread or white rice.

- 3.Add healthy fats: Healthy fats are essential for brain function and hormone production. Include sources such as avocados, nuts and seeds, olive oil, or fatty fish like salmon in your meals.

- 4.Don't forget about fruits and vegetables: Fruits and vegetables are packed with vitamins, minerals, fiber, and antioxidants that support overall health. Aim to fill half your plate with colorful fruits and vegetables to ensure an adequate intake of these vital nutrients.

- 5.Be mindful of portion sizes: While it's important to include a variety of nutrient-rich foods in your meals, it's equally important to be mindful of portion sizes.Gorging can prompt weight gain and other medical problems. Utilize more modest plates and bowls, and pay attention to your body's appetite and completion signs.

By creating balanced meals with a variety of nutrient-rich foods, you can ensure that your body is receiving the necessary nutrients for optimal health and well-being. Experiment with different recipes and flavors to keep your meals interesting and enjoyable.

6.2 Portion Control and Mindful Eating

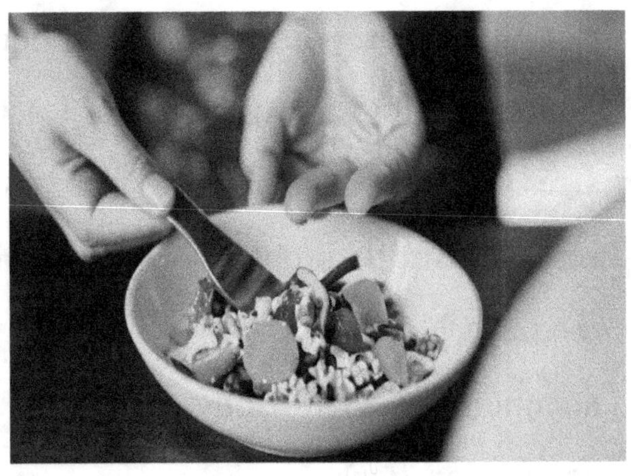

Portion control and mindful eating are crucial aspects of meal planning for optimal nutrition. In today's society, where large portion sizes have become the norm, it is easy to consume more calories than our bodies actually need. This can lead to weight gain and an increased risk of chronic diseases such as diabetes and heart disease.

Practicing portion control involves being aware of how much food you are consuming and adjusting your portions accordingly. Here are some strategies to help you practice portion control:

- 1.Use measuring cups or a food scale:

  Measuring cups or a food scale can help

you accurately measure serving sizes, especially when cooking at home. This ensures that you are not unknowingly consuming larger portions than recommended.

- 2.Read food labels: Pay attention to serving sizes listed on food labels. Many packaged foods contain multiple servings per container, so be mindful of how much you are actually consuming.

- 3.Fill half your plate with vegetables: By filling half your plate with vegetables, you automatically reduce the space available for higher-calorie foods. This helps control portion sizes while still providing essential nutrients.

- 4.Slow down and savor each bite: Mindful eating involves paying attention to the taste, texture, and aroma of each bite of food. By slowing down and savoring each bite, you give your brain time to register feelings of fullness, preventing overeating.

- 5.Listen to your body's hunger cues: Eat when you're hungry and stop when you're satisfied, not when you're overly full. Tune in to your body's hunger and fullness cues to avoid mindless eating.

Practicing portion control and mindful eating can help you maintain a healthy weight, prevent overeating, and improve digestion. By being aware of your portion sizes and listening to your body's signals, you can develop a healthier relationship with food.

6.3 Incorporating Superfoods into Your Diet

Incorporating superfoods into your diet is an excellent way to boost the nutritional value of your meals. Superfoods supplement thick food sources that are plentiful in nutrients, minerals, cell reinforcements, and other helpful mixtures. They have been shown to provide numerous health benefits, including reducing inflammation, improving heart health, boosting immunity, and supporting brain function.

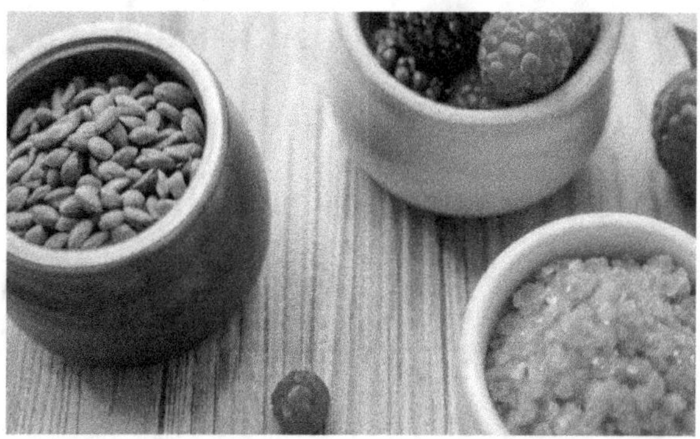

Here are some popular superfoods that you can incorporate into your diet:

- 1.Berries: Berries such as blueberries, strawberries, and raspberries are packed with antioxidants that help protect against oxidative stress and reduce the risk of chronic diseases like cancer and heart disease. Add them to smoothies, yogurt bowls, or enjoy them as a snack.

- 2.Leafy greens: Leafy greens like spinach, kale, and Swiss chard are loaded with vitamins A, C, K, and folate. They also contain fiber and various minerals such as iron and calcium. Include them in salads or sauté them as a side dish for added nutrition.

- 3.Salmon: Salmon is an excellent source of omega-3 fatty acids that support heart health and brain function. It is also rich in high-quality protein. Barbecue or prepare salmon filets for a delightful and nutritious feast.

- 4.Chia seeds: Chia seeds are packed with fiber, omega-3 fatty acids, protein, calcium, magnesium, and antioxidants. They can be added to smoothies or used as a topping for yogurt or oatmeal for an extra nutritional boost.

- 5.Quinoa: Quinoa is a gluten-free grain that is high in protein, fiber, and various vitamins and minerals. It can be used as a base for salads, added to soups, or served as a side dish.

- 6.Turmeric: Turmeric contains a compound called curcumin, which has powerful anti-inflammatory and antioxidant properties. Add turmeric to curries, smoothies, or golden milk for its health benefits.

Incorporating superfoods into your diet doesn't have to be complicated or expensive. Start by adding one or two superfoods at a time and gradually increase the variety. Experiment with different recipes and find creative ways to include these nutrient powerhouses in your meals.

By incorporating superfoods into your diet, you can enhance the nutritional value of your meals and support overall health and well-being. Remember that while superfoods offer numerous health benefits, they should be part of a balanced diet that includes a variety of other nutrient-rich foods as well.

In conclusion, creating balanced meals with a variety of nutrient-rich foods, practicing portion control and mindful eating, and incorporating superfoods into your diet are all essential components of meal planning for optimal nutrition. By following these strategies, you can ensure that you are providing your body with the necessary nutrients it needs to thrive. Make sure to stand by listening to your body's signals and pursue decisions that line up with your singular requirements and inclinations. Start implementing these practices today and embark on a journey towards better nutrition and improved overall health.

Chapter 7

Special Considerations for Different Lifestyles

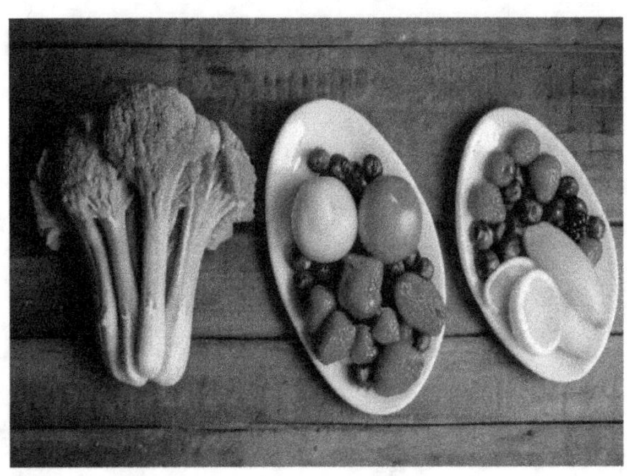

7.1 Vegetarianism and Veganism: Meeting Nutritional Needs without Animal Products

Vegetarianism and veganism have become increasingly popular lifestyles for various reasons, including ethical concerns, environmental sustainability, and health benefits. However, eliminating animal products from the diet requires careful planning to ensure that all essential nutrients are obtained.

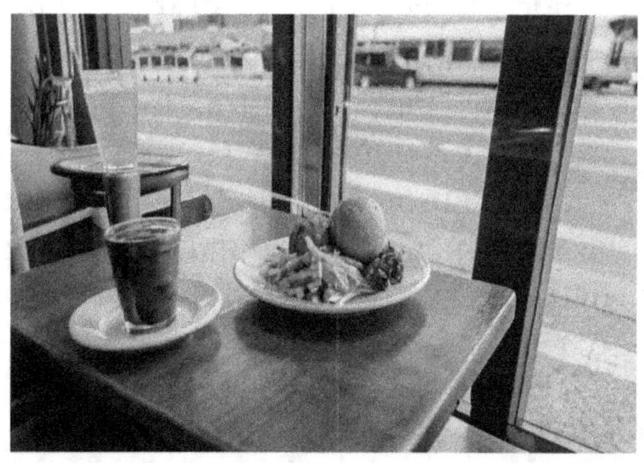

One of the main concerns for vegetarians and vegans is meeting their protein needs. While animal products are complete sources of protein, plant-based sources can also provide all the necessary amino acids when combined properly. For example, combining legumes with grains or seeds can create a complete protein profile. Quinoa with black beans or peanut butter on whole wheat bread are excellent examples of such combinations.

Iron is another nutrient that may require special attention in vegetarian and vegan diets. Plant-based iron sources, known as non-heme iron, are not as easily absorbed by the body compared to heme iron found in animal products. To enhance absorption, it is recommended to consume vitamin C-rich foods alongside iron-rich plant foods. For instance, pairing spinach salad with citrus fruits or adding bell peppers to a lentil stew can significantly increase iron absorption.Omega-3 unsaturated fats are fundamental for mind wellbeing and decreasing irritation in the body.

While fish is a common source of omega-3s, vegetarians and vegans can obtain these fatty acids from plant-based sources such as flaxseeds, chia seeds, walnuts, and algae-based supplements. Including these foods regularly in the diet ensures an adequate intake of omega-3s.

Calcium is often associated with dairy products; however, there are plenty of plant-based sources that provide this essential mineral. Dark leafy greens like kale and broccoli are excellent calcium sources. Additionally, fortified plant milks and tofu made with calcium sulfate can contribute to meeting daily calcium requirements.

Vitamin B12 is exclusively found in animal products, making it a crucial nutrient for vegetarians and vegans to pay attention to. It is recommended to include fortified foods or take B12 supplements to ensure adequate intake. Regular blood tests can also help monitor B12 levels and determine if supplementation is necessary.

By incorporating a variety of plant-based foods and paying attention to nutrient combinations, vegetarians and vegans can meet their nutritional needs without relying on animal products. It is important to consult with a registered dietitian or nutritionist who specializes in plant-based diets to ensure proper guidance and support.

7.2 Sports Nutrition: Fueling Performance and Recovery

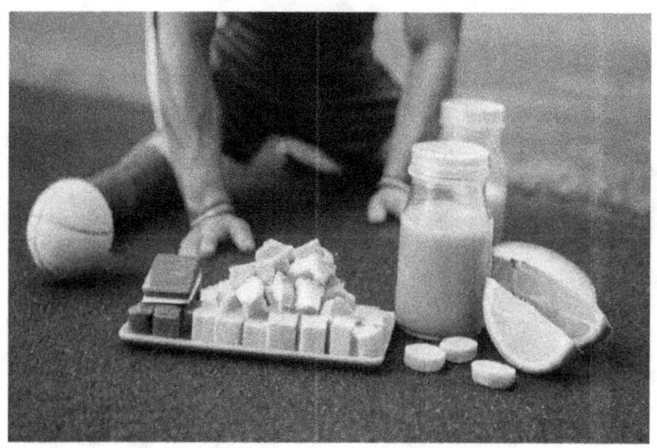

Sports nutrition plays a vital role in optimizing athletic performance, improving recuperation, and supporting generally speaking wellbeing. Competitors have special healthful necessities because of the actual requests put on their bodies during preparation and contest. Proper fueling before, during, and after exercise is essential for maximizing performance.

Carbohydrates are the primary source of energy for athletes as they provide readily available fuel for muscles. Complex carbohydrates like whole grains, fruits, vegetables, and legumes should form the foundation of an athlete's diet. These foods provide sustained energy release and are rich in vitamins, minerals, and fiber.

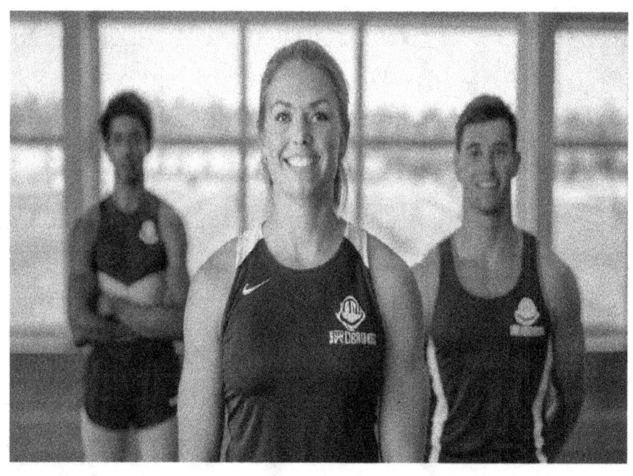

Protein is crucial for muscle repair and growth. Athletes require slightly more protein than sedentary individuals to support their training regimen. Good sources of protein include lean meats, poultry, fish, dairy products, eggs, legumes, nuts, seeds, and soy products. Distributing protein intake evenly throughout the day helps optimize muscle protein synthesis.

Hydration is one more basic part of sports nourishment. Lack of hydration can hinder execution and increment the gamble of intensity related diseases. Athletes should aim to drink fluids regularly throughout the day and consume additional fluids before, during, and after exercise. Water is usually sufficient for most activities; however, prolonged intense exercise may require electrolyte-rich beverages or sports drinks.

Timing meals appropriately around training sessions is essential for optimal performance. Consuming a balanced meal or snack containing carbohydrates and protein 2-3 hours before exercise provides the necessary energy and nutrients. During prolonged endurance activities, consuming easily digestible carbohydrates such as sports gels or drinks can help maintain blood sugar levels and delay fatigue.

Post-exercise nutrition is crucial for recovery and muscle glycogen replenishment. Consuming a combination of carbohydrates and protein within 30 minutes to an hour after exercise helps kick start the recovery process. This can be achieved through a post-workout shake, a balanced meal, or snacks like Greek yogurt with fruit or a peanut butter sandwich.

Supplements can be beneficial in certain situations, but they should not replace whole foods. Athletes should focus on meeting their nutritional needs through a well-balanced diet first. However, some supplements like creatine, beta-alanine, and caffeine have been shown to enhance performance in specific sports when used appropriately under professional guidance.

It is important for athletes to work with registered dietitians who specialize in sports nutrition to develop personalized plans that meet their unique needs. These professionals can provide guidance on nutrient timing, portion sizes, hydration strategies, and supplement use based on individual goals and training demands.

7.3 Pregnancy and Breastfeeding: Ensuring Adequate Nutrition for Mother and Baby

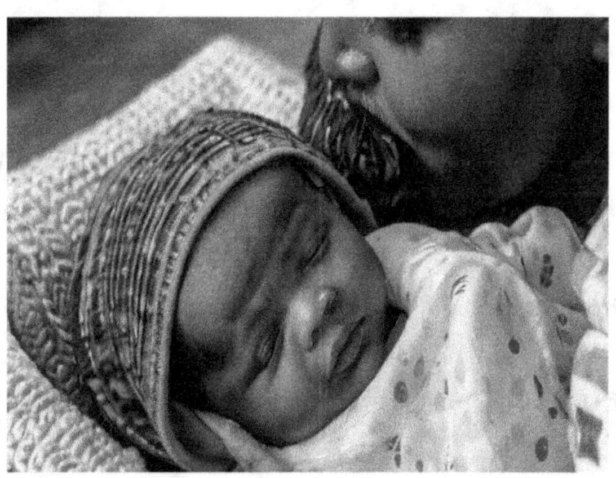

Pregnancy is a time of increased nutritional needs to support the growth and development of both the mother and the baby. Proper nutrition during pregnancy plays a crucial role in ensuring a healthy pregnancy, reducing the risk of complications, and supporting fetal development.

During pregnancy, it is important to consume additional calories to meet the increased energy demands. However, these extra calories should come from nutrient-dense foods rather than empty calories from sugary snacks or processed foods. Focusing on whole grains, lean proteins, fruits, vegetables, dairy products or plant-based alternatives ensures an adequate intake of essential nutrients.

Folic acid is one of the most important nutrients during pregnancy as it helps prevent neural tube defects in the developing baby. It is recommended to consume foods rich in folate, such as leafy greens, legumes, fortified cereals, and citrus fruits. In some cases, a folic acid supplement may be prescribed by healthcare providers.

Iron is essential for the production of red blood cells and oxygen transport. Pregnant women often require additional iron to support the increased blood volume and meet the needs of the growing fetus. Good sources of iron include lean meats, poultry, fish, legumes, fortified cereals, and dark leafy greens. Consuming vitamin C-rich foods alongside iron-rich foods enhances absorption.

Calcium is crucial for fetal bone development and maintaining maternal bone health. Dairy products or plant-based alternatives like fortified plant milks are excellent sources of calcium. Adequate vitamin D intake is also important for calcium absorption; therefore, spending time outdoors or taking a vitamin D supplement may be necessary.

Omega-3 fatty acids are vital for brain and eye development in the fetus. Consuming fatty fish like salmon or trout twice a week can provide an adequate intake of omega-3s. For those who do not consume fish due to dietary preferences or concerns about mercury levels, algae-based supplements can be a suitable alternative.

Proper hydration is essential during pregnancy to support blood volume expansion and prevent constipation. Pregnant women should aim to drink plenty of fluids throughout the day and listen to their body's thirst cues.

Breastfeeding mothers have unique nutritional needs as they provide all the nutrients for their infants through breast milk. It is important for breastfeeding mothers to consume an additional 500 calories per day compared to their pre-pregnancy needs. A well-balanced diet that includes whole grains, lean proteins, fruits, vegetables, dairy products or plant-based alternatives ensures an adequate nutrient supply for both mother and baby.

In conclusion, vegetarianism and veganism require careful planning to meet nutritional needs without animal products. Sports nutrition plays a vital role in fueling performance and recovery for athletes. Pregnancy and breastfeeding require special attention to ensure adequate nutrition for both the mother and baby. By understanding these special considerations, individuals can make informed choices to support their unique lifestyles and nutritional needs.

Chapter 8

Nutrition for Specific Health Conditions

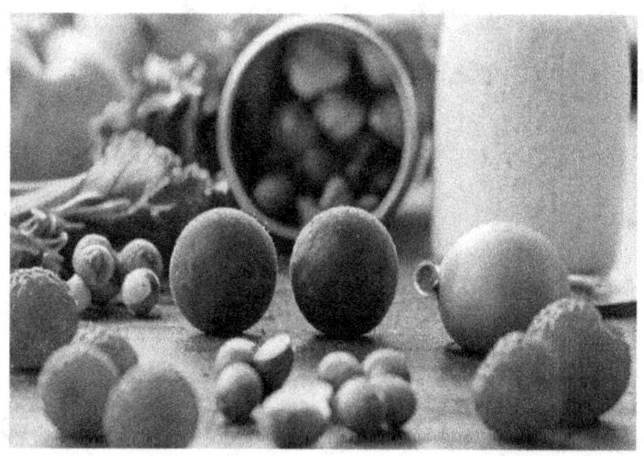

8.1 Heart-Healthy Diet: Lowering Cholesterol and Blood Pressure

A heart-healthy diet is crucial for maintaining cardiovascular health and reducing the risk of heart disease. One of the key components of a heart-healthy diet is lowering cholesterol levels and blood pressure. High cholesterol levels and elevated blood pressure are major risk factors for heart disease, so it is important to address these issues through proper nutrition.

To lower cholesterol levels, it is essential to reduce the intake of saturated fats and trans fats. These unhealthy fats can raise LDL (bad) cholesterol levels in the blood, leading to plaque buildup in the arteries. Instead, focus on consuming healthy fats such as monounsaturated fats found in olive oil, avocados, and nuts, as well as polyunsaturated fats found in fatty fish like salmon and trout.

In addition to reducing unhealthy fats, increasing dietary fiber intake can also help lower cholesterol levels. Soluble fiber found in foods like oats, barley, legumes, and fruits can bind to cholesterol in the digestive system and prevent its absorption into the bloodstream. This can effectively reduce LDL cholesterol levels.

Another important aspect of a heart-healthy diet is managing blood pressure. High blood pressure puts strain on the arteries and increases the risk of heart disease. To control blood pressure through diet, it is crucial to limit sodium intake. Sodium can cause fluid retention in the body, leading to increased blood volume and higher blood pressure. Avoiding processed foods that are high in sodium and opting for fresh ingredients instead can significantly reduce sodium intake.

Potassium-rich foods should also be incorporated into a heart-healthy diet as they help counteract the effects of sodium on blood pressure. Foods such as bananas, oranges, spinach, sweet potatoes, and yogurt are excellent sources of potassium.

Furthermore, adopting the DASH (Dietary Approaches to Stop Hypertension) eating plan has been shown to effectively lower blood pressure. The DASH diet emphasizes fruits, vegetables, whole grains, lean proteins, and low-fat dairy products while limiting saturated fats, cholesterol, and sodium. Following this eating plan can not only help lower blood pressure but also improve overall cardiovascular health.

Real-world examples of individuals who have successfully implemented a heart-healthy diet to lower cholesterol and blood pressure can be inspiring. For instance, John, a middle-aged man with high cholesterol and hypertension, decided to make significant changes to his diet. He eliminated processed foods from his meals and focused on consuming whole foods rich in healthy fats and fiber. He incorporated regular exercise into his routine as well. After a few months of following this heart-healthy lifestyle, John's cholesterol levels decreased significantly, and his blood pressure returned to normal range.

In conclusion, adopting a heart-healthy diet is crucial for lowering cholesterol levels and blood pressure. By reducing the intake of unhealthy fats, increasing dietary fiber consumption, limiting sodium intake, incorporating potassium-rich foods, and following the DASH eating plan, individuals can effectively improve their cardiovascular health. Real-life success stories like John's demonstrate the positive impact that a heart-healthy diet can have on overall well-being.

8.2 Diabetes Management: Controlling Blood Sugar Levels through Diet

Diabetes is a chronic condition characterized by high blood sugar levels due to the body's inability to produce or properly use insulin.

Proper nutrition plays a vital role in managing diabetes by controlling blood sugar levels. A well-balanced diet that focuses on portion control and includes nutrient-dense foods can help individuals with diabetes maintain stable blood sugar levels.

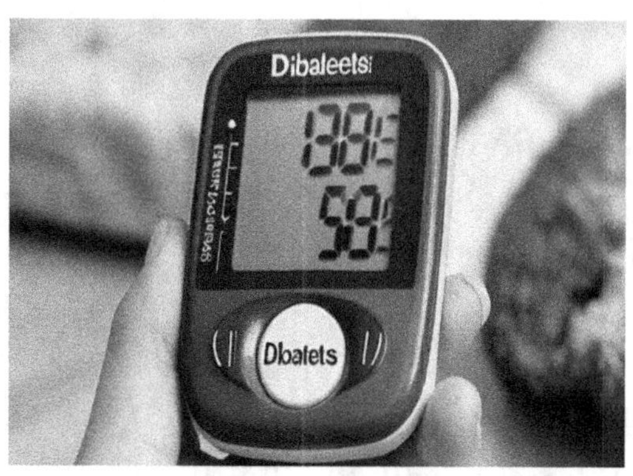

One of the key principles of managing diabetes through diet is monitoring carbohydrate intake. Carbohydrates directly affect blood sugar levels as they are broken down into glucose during digestion. It is important for individuals with diabetes to choose carbohydrates wisely and distribute them evenly throughout the day to prevent spikes in blood sugar.

Foods with a low glycemic index (GI) are recommended for individuals with diabetes as they cause a slower and more gradual rise in blood sugar levels. Instances of low GI food sources incorporate entire grains, vegetables, non-bland vegetables, and most natural products. These foods provide a steady release of glucose into the bloodstream, preventing sudden spikes in blood sugar.

In addition to choosing the right carbohydrates, portion control is crucial for managing diabetes. Controlling portion sizes helps regulate calorie intake and prevents excessive blood sugar fluctuations. Measuring food portions using tools such as measuring cups or a food scale can be helpful in maintaining consistency.

Another important aspect of diabetes management is including lean proteins in meals. Protein-rich foods like poultry, fish, tofu, and legumes have minimal impact on blood sugar levels and can help promote satiety. Including protein in each meal can also slow down the digestion of carbohydrates, leading to a more gradual release of glucose into the bloodstream.

Furthermore, healthy fats should be incorporated into a diabetes-friendly diet. Unsaturated fats found in avocados, nuts, seeds, and olive oil can help improve insulin sensitivity and reduce the risk of heart disease often associated with diabetes. However, it is important to consume these fats in moderation due to their high calorie content.

Real-life examples of individuals successfully managing their diabetes through diet can provide inspiration for others facing similar challenges. For instance, Sarah was diagnosed with type 2 diabetes and struggled to control her blood sugar levels initially. She decided to adopt a low-carbohydrate diet that focused on whole foods and limited processed sugars and refined grains. By monitoring her carbohydrate intake carefully and incorporating regular exercise into her routine, Sarah was able to achieve stable blood sugar levels over time.

In conclusion, controlling blood sugar levels through diet is essential for managing diabetes effectively. By monitoring carbohydrate intake, practicing portion control, including lean proteins in meals, incorporating healthy fats moderately, and choosing low GI foods, individuals with diabetes can maintain stable blood sugar levels and improve their overall well-being. Real-life success stories like Sarah's demonstrate the positive impact that a diabetes-friendly diet can have on managing the condition.

8.3 Weight Management: Achieving a Healthy Body Weight through Nutrition.

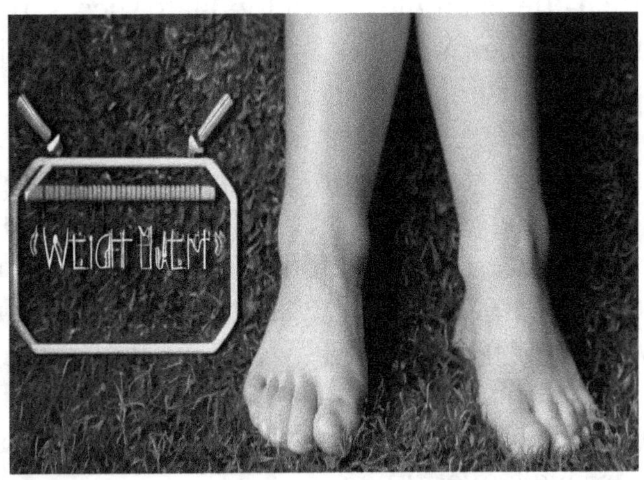

Weight management is a common concern for many individuals, as maintaining a healthy body weight is crucial for overall health and well-being. Proper nutrition plays a key role in achieving and maintaining a healthy weight. By focusing on nutrient-dense foods, practicing portion control, and adopting sustainable eating habits, individuals can effectively manage their weight.

One of the fundamental principles of weight management is consuming nutrient-dense foods. Nutrient-dense foods are rich in essential vitamins, minerals, and other beneficial compounds while being relatively low in calories. These foods provide the body with the necessary nutrients without excessive calorie intake. Instances of supplement thick food varieties incorporate natural products, vegetables, entire grains, lean proteins, and low-fat dairy items.

In addition to choosing nutrient-dense foods, portion control is essential for weight management. It is important to be mindful of serving sizes and avoid overeating. Using smaller plates or bowls can help create an illusion of larger portions while reducing actual calorie intake.

Another effective strategy for weight management is adopting sustainable eating habits rather than relying on restrictive diets or quick fixes. Sustainable eating habits focus on long-term lifestyle changes rather than short-term solutions. This includes listening to hunger cues, practicing mindful eating, and developing a balanced relationship with food.

Regular physical activity also plays a crucial role in weight management alongside proper nutrition. Engaging in regular exercise helps burn calories, build muscle mass, increase metabolism, and improve overall fitness levels. Combining regular physical activity with a balanced diet creates an effective approach to achieving and maintaining a healthy body weight.

Real-world examples of individuals who have successfully managed their weight through nutrition can be inspiring for others seeking similar goals. For instance, Lisa struggled with her weight for years but decided to make sustainable changes to her eating habits. She focused on consuming nutrient-dense foods, practiced portion control, and incorporated regular exercise into her routine. Over time, Lisa achieved a healthy body weight and improved her overall well-being.

In conclusion, achieving a healthy body weight through nutrition requires focusing on nutrient-dense foods, practicing portion control, adopting sustainable eating habits, and incorporating regular physical activity. By making these lifestyle changes, individuals can effectively manage their weight and improve their overall health. Real-life success stories like Lisa's demonstrate the positive impact that proper nutrition can have on achieving weight management goals.

Chapter 9

Nutritional Supplements

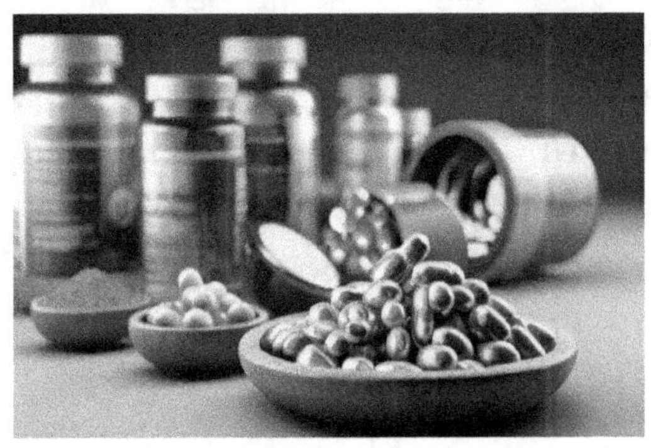

9.1 Understanding the Role of Supplements in Meeting Nutritional Needs

Supplements play a crucial role in meeting our nutritional needs, especially when our diet falls short in providing all the essential nutrients our body requires. While it is always best to obtain nutrients from whole foods, there are certain situations where supplements can be beneficial.

One such situation is when an individual has specific dietary restrictions or preferences that limit their intake of certain nutrients. For example, vegetarians and vegans may struggle to get enough vitamin B12, which is primarily found in animal products. In such cases, a B12 supplement can help bridge the gap and ensure adequate intake.

Additionally, some individuals may have medical conditions or undergo treatments that affect nutrient absorption or increase nutrient requirements. For instance, people with celiac disease may have difficulty absorbing nutrients from food due to damage to their small intestine. In these cases, supplements can provide the necessary vitamins and minerals that may otherwise be lacking.

Furthermore, supplements can be particularly useful for athletes and individuals with high physical activity levels. Intense exercise increases nutrient demands, and supplements like protein powders or amino acid supplements can aid in muscle recovery and growth.

It's important to note that while supplements can be beneficial in certain situations, they should not replace a balanced diet. Whole foods contain a wide array of nutrients that work synergistically together, providing benefits beyond what individual supplements can offer. Therefore, it is always recommended to prioritize whole foods as the primary source of nutrition and use supplements as a complement when necessary.

To better understand the role of supplements in meeting nutritional needs, let's consider an example. Imagine a busy professional who often relies on fast food for meals due to time constraints. This person's diet lacks essential vitamins and minerals found abundantly in fruits and vegetables. By incorporating a multivitamin supplement into their routine, they can ensure they are getting at least some of the necessary nutrients that their diet is lacking. However, it's important for this individual to also make an effort to include more whole foods in their diet to achieve optimal nutrition.

9.2 Evaluating the Safety and Efficacy of Different Supplements

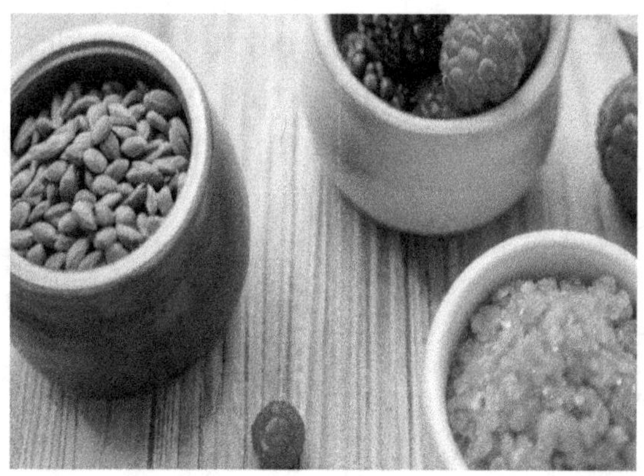

When considering supplements, it is crucial to evaluate their safety and efficacy before incorporating them into your routine. Not all supplements are created equal, and some may have potential risks or lack scientific evidence supporting their effectiveness.

One way to ensure the safety of a supplement is by looking for third-party certifications or seals of approval on the product packaging. These certifications indicate that the supplement has undergone rigorous testing and meets certain quality standards. Examples of reputable certifications include NSF International, United States Pharmacopeia (USP), and ConsumerLab.com.

Another important aspect to consider is the scientific evidence supporting the efficacy of a supplement. Look for supplements that have been studied extensively in well-designed clinical trials with human subjects. Peer-reviewed research articles published in reputable scientific journals are good indicators of a supplement's effectiveness.

It's also essential to be cautious of exaggerated claims or promises made by supplement manufacturers. On the off chance that an item appears to be unrealistic, it likely is. Be skeptical of supplements that claim to cure diseases or offer miraculous results without any scientific evidence backing them up.

To illustrate the importance of evaluating supplements, let's consider the example of weight loss supplements. Many products on the market claim to help individuals shed pounds effortlessly. However, upon closer examination, most of these supplements lack substantial scientific evidence supporting their effectiveness. In fact, some weight loss supplements have been found to contain harmful ingredients or have adverse side effects. Therefore, it is crucial to do thorough research and consult with healthcare professionals before using any weight loss supplement.

By critically evaluating the safety and efficacy of different supplements, individuals can make informed decisions about which ones are worth incorporating into their routine.

9.3 Choosing the Right Supplements for Your Individual Needs

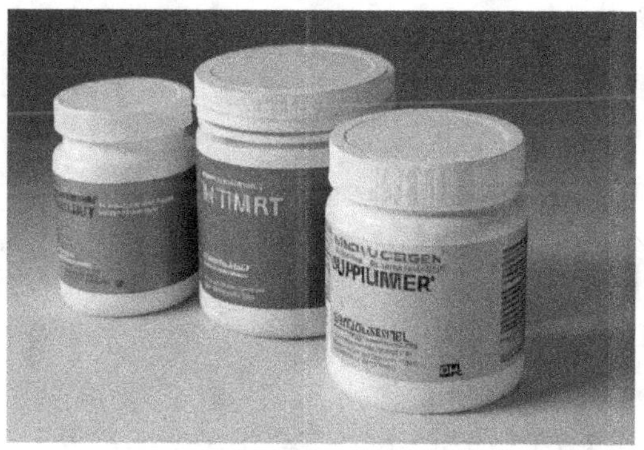

Choosing the right supplements for your individual needs requires careful consideration of various factors, including your specific nutritional requirements, health conditions, and lifestyle.

First and foremost, it is essential to identify any nutrient deficiencies or imbalances that may exist. This can be done through blood tests or by consulting with a healthcare professional. Once you have a clear understanding of which nutrients you may be lacking, you can select supplements that target those specific deficiencies.

Consider your overall health status and any existing medical conditions when choosing supplements. Certain health conditions may require specific nutrients or necessitate avoiding certain supplements altogether. For example, individuals with kidney disease may need to limit their intake of certain minerals like potassium or phosphorus.

Additionally, take into account your lifestyle and dietary preferences. If you follow a vegetarian or vegan diet, you may need to consider supplements like vitamin B12 or iron. Athletes or individuals with high physical activity levels may benefit from protein powders or branched-chain amino acid (BCAA) supplements to support muscle recovery and growth.

It's also important to consider the form and dosage of the supplement. Some nutrients are better absorbed in certain forms than others.For instance, calcium citrate is more effortlessly consumed than calcium carbonate. Additionally, pay attention to the recommended dosage and ensure it aligns with your individual needs.

To illustrate the process of choosing the right supplements for individual needs, let's consider an example of someone who follows a plant-based diet and has been experiencing low energy levels. After consulting with a healthcare professional and conducting blood tests, they discover they have low iron levels due to inadequate intake from plant-based sources alone. In this case, they can choose an iron supplement specifically formulated for better absorption in non-heme iron sources commonly found in plants.

In conclusion, choosing the right supplements for your individual needs requires careful consideration of factors such as nutrient deficiencies, health conditions, lifestyle, and dietary preferences. By taking these factors into account and consulting with healthcare professionals, individuals can make informed decisions about which supplements are most suitable for them. Remember, supplements should always be used as a complement to a balanced diet and not as a replacement for whole foods.

Chapter 10

Practical Tips for Incorporating Optimal Nutrition into Your Lifestyle

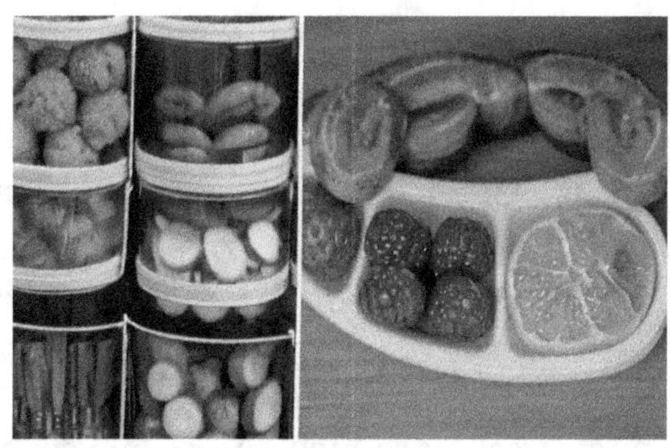

10.1 Grocery Shopping Strategies for Nutrient-Dense Foods

When it comes to optimizing your nutrition, one of the most important steps is grocery shopping. By selecting nutrient-dense foods at the store, you can ensure that your meals are packed with essential vitamins, minerals, and other beneficial compounds. Here are some strategies to help you make the most out of your grocery shopping experience:

- 1.Plan Ahead: Before heading to the store, take some time to plan your meals for the week. This won't just set aside your time and cash yet additionally assist you with pursuing better decisions. Create a shopping list based on your planned meals and stick to it as much as possible.

- 2.Shop the Perimeter: The perimeter of the grocery store is usually where you'll find fresh produce, lean meats, dairy products, and whole grains. These are typically more nutrient-dense options compared to processed foods found in the aisles. Focus on filling your cart with fruits, vegetables, lean proteins like chicken or fish, and whole grains like quinoa or brown rice.

- 3.Read Labels Carefully: While shopping for packaged foods, it's crucial to read labels carefully. Search for items that have negligible added sugars, undesirable fats, and counterfeit fixings. Pay attention to serving sizes as well to ensure you're getting an accurate understanding of what you're consuming.

- 4.Choose Colorful Produce: When selecting fruits and vegetables, opt for a variety of colors. Different colors indicate different nutrients present in these foods. For example, orange fruits like oranges and carrots are rich in vitamin C and beta-carotene while leafy greens like spinach are packed with iron and folate.

- 5.Buy in Bulk: Buying certain items in bulk can be cost-effective and convenient. Staples like whole grains (oats, quinoa), nuts/seeds (almonds, chia seeds), and legumes (lentils, chickpeas) can be purchased in larger quantities and stored for longer periods. This way, you'll always have nutrient-dense options on hand.

- 6.Consider Frozen and Canned Options: Don't overlook frozen or canned fruits and vegetables. These can be just as nutritious as fresh produce, especially when they are picked at their peak ripeness and immediately frozen or canned. They are also convenient to have on hand for quick meals or snacks.

- 7.Shop Locally and Seasonally: Whenever possible, support local farmers by shopping at farmers' markets or joining a community-supported agriculture (CSA) program. Locally grown produce is often fresher and more nutrient-dense since it doesn't have to travel long distances. Additionally, buying seasonal produce ensures that you're getting the most flavorful and nutritious options available.

By implementing these grocery shopping strategies, you can make informed choices that prioritize nutrient-dense foods. Remember that small changes in your shopping habits can lead to significant improvements in your overall nutrition.

10.2 Cooking Techniques to Preserve Nutrients in Food

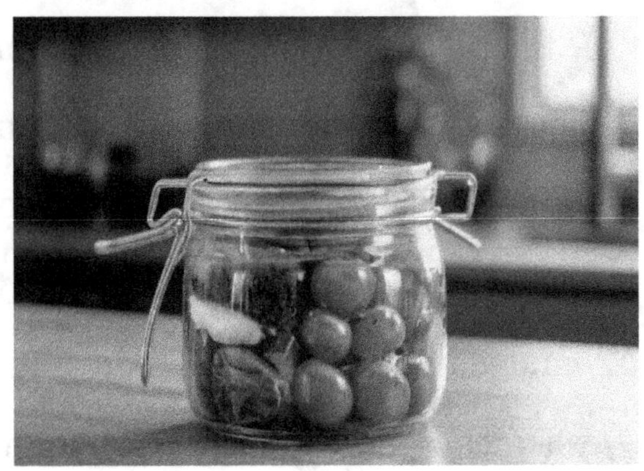

Cooking is not only a way to prepare food but also an opportunity to maximize the nutritional value of the ingredients you use. While some nutrients may be lost during cooking, there are several techniques you can employ to preserve as many nutrients as possible:

- 1.Use Minimal Water: When boiling vegetables or grains, use the minimum amount of water necessary. Excessive water can cause water-soluble vitamins like vitamin C and B vitamins to leach out into the cooking liquid. Steaming or sautéing vegetables with a small amount of oil can help retain more nutrients.

- 2.Cook at Lower Temperatures: High heat can degrade certain nutrients, so it's best to cook foods at lower temperatures whenever possible. For example, roasting vegetables at a moderate temperature rather than frying them at high heat helps preserve their nutrient content.

- 3.Preserve Cooking Liquid: When you cook foods like vegetables or legumes, save the cooking liquid and incorporate it into soups, stews, or sauces. This liquid contains water-soluble vitamins and minerals that would otherwise be lost if discarded.

- 4.Opt for Quick Cooking Methods: The longer you cook food, the more nutrients are likely to be lost. Quick cooking methods like stir-frying or blanching can help retain more nutrients compared to prolonged boiling or baking.

- 5.Store Cut Vegetables Properly: If you're prepping vegetables in advance, store them properly to minimize nutrient loss. Exposure to air and light can cause oxidation and nutrient degradation. Keep cut vegetables in airtight containers in the refrigerator until ready to use.

- 6.Add Acidic Ingredients: Adding acidic ingredients like lemon juice or vinegar to your dishes can help preserve certain nutrients. For example, vitamin C is sensitive to heat but can be stabilized by adding lemon juice to cooked vegetables.

- 7.Don't Overcook Proteins: Overcooking proteins like meat or fish can lead to nutrient loss and decreased digestibility. Cook proteins until they are just done rather than well-done to retain as many nutrients as possible.

By employing these cooking techniques, you can ensure that your meals are not only delicious but also packed with essential nutrients. Experiment with different methods and find what works best for you while keeping nutrition at the forefront of your culinary endeavors.

10.3 Eating Out and Traveling while Maintaining a Balanced Diet

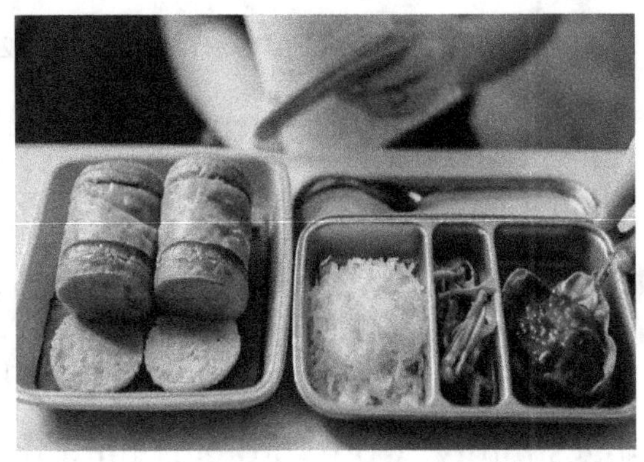

Maintaining a balanced diet doesn't have to be challenging when eating out or traveling. With some planning and mindful choices, you can still enjoy delicious meals while prioritizing your nutritional needs:

- 1.Research Restaurants in Advance: Before dining out, take some time to research restaurants in the area you'll be visiting or where you plan on eating out locally. Look for establishments that offer healthier options or cater to specific dietary needs. Many restaurants now provide their menus online, allowing you to assess the available choices beforehand.

- 2.Make Special Requests: Don't be afraid to make special requests when ordering at a restaurant. Ask for dressings or sauces on the side, substitute fries for a side salad or steamed vegetables, and request grilled or baked options instead of fried ones. Most restaurants are accommodating and willing to make adjustments to meet your dietary preferences.

- 3.Practice Portion Control: Restaurant portions tend to be larger than what we need for a single meal. Consider sharing an entrée with a dining partner or ask for a takeout container at the beginning of the meal and pack up half of your dish before you start eating. This way, you can enjoy your meal without overindulging.

- 4.Choose Nutrient-Dense Options: Look for menu items that are rich in nutrients rather than empty calories. Opt for dishes that include lean proteins like grilled chicken or fish, whole grains like quinoa or brown rice, and plenty of vegetables. Avoid deep-fried foods and opt for steamed, roasted, or grilled options instead.

- 5.Stay Hydrated: It's easy to forget about hydration while traveling or dining out, but it's essential for maintaining overall health and well-being. Carry a reusable water bottle with you and drink water throughout the day to stay hydrated and avoid unnecessary sugary beverages.

- 6.Pack Healthy Snacks: When traveling, it's always a good idea to pack some healthy snacks in case you find yourself hungry between meals or unable to find nutritious options easily. Nuts, seeds, dried fruits, granola bars, and fresh fruit are all portable snack options that can help keep you fueled throughout your journey.

- 7.Be Mindful of Alcohol Consumption: Alcoholic beverages can add empty calories and hinder your ability to make mindful food choices while dining out or traveling. Limit alcohol consumption and opt for healthier alternatives like sparkling water with a splash of fruit juice or herbal tea.

Remember, maintaining a balanced diet is about making conscious choices and finding the best options available to you. By planning ahead, making special requests, and being mindful of your choices, you can enjoy eating out and traveling while still prioritizing your nutritional needs.

Incorporating optimal nutrition into your lifestyle doesn't have to be overwhelming. By implementing these practical tips for grocery shopping, cooking techniques, and dining out/traveling, you can make significant strides towards achieving a balanced diet. Remember that small changes in your habits can lead to long-term improvements in your overall health and well-being. Start incorporating these strategies today and embark on a journey towards better nutrition!

Chapter 11

Conclusion and Next Steps

11.1 Recap of Key Concepts and Takeaways

In this final chapter, we will recap the key concepts and takeaways from our comprehensive guide on achieving optimal nutrition. Throughout this book, we have explored various aspects of nutrition, including macronutrients, micronutrients, meal planning, and portion control. By understanding these key concepts, you can make informed choices about your diet and ensure that you are getting all the essential nutrients your body needs.

One of the main takeaways from this guide is the importance of a balanced diet. A balanced diet consists of a variety of foods from different food groups to provide all the necessary nutrients. It is crucial to include carbohydrates, proteins, fats, vitamins, minerals, and water in your daily meals to support overall health and well-being.

Another key concept is the role of macronutrients in our diet. Macronutrients include carbohydrates, proteins, and fats, which are essential for energy production and various bodily functions. Understanding the sources and functions of these macronutrients can help you make healthier choices when it comes to selecting foods for your meals.

Micronutrients are similarly significant however expected in more modest amounts contrasted with macronutrients. These include vitamins and minerals that play vital roles in maintaining good health. By incorporating a variety of fruits, vegetables, whole grains, lean meats, dairy products or alternatives into your diet, you can ensure an adequate intake of micronutrients.

Meal planning is another crucial aspect covered in this guide. Planning your meals in advance allows you to make healthier choices and avoid impulsive decisions based on convenience or cravings. By creating a weekly meal plan that includes a balance of macronutrients and incorporates a variety of foods from different food groups, you can sustain optimal nutrition over the long term.

Portion control is also emphasized throughout this guide as it plays a significant role in maintaining a healthy weight and preventing overeating. Understanding appropriate portion sizes and practicing mindful eating can help you avoid consuming excess calories and maintain a balanced diet.

Lastly, we have discussed the importance of hydration in achieving optimal nutrition. Water is fundamental for different physical processes, including assimilation, supplement retention, and waste disposal. Staying hydrated throughout the day is crucial for maintaining overall health and well-being.

By incorporating these key concepts into your daily life, you can make significant strides towards achieving optimal nutrition and improving your overall health.

11.2 Developing a Long-Term Plan for Sustaining Optimal Nutrition

Now that you have gained a comprehensive understanding of nutrition and its importance, it is essential to develop a long-term plan for sustaining optimal nutrition. While short-term changes in your diet can yield immediate benefits, it is crucial to adopt sustainable habits that will support your nutritional goals in the long run.

One effective strategy for sustaining optimal nutrition is setting realistic goals. Start by identifying specific areas of your diet that need improvement and set achievable targets. For example, if you want to increase your vegetable intake, aim to include at least one serving of vegetables with each meal. By setting small, attainable goals, you are more likely to stay motivated and maintain consistency.

Another important aspect of sustaining optimal nutrition is creating a supportive environment. Surround yourself with people who share similar health goals or seek out online communities where you can find support and encouragement. Having a support system can make it easier to stick to your nutritional plan and overcome any challenges or setbacks along the way.

Meal prepping is another valuable tool for sustaining optimal nutrition. By dedicating some time each week to prepare meals in advance, you can ensure that healthy options are readily available when hunger strikes. This not only saves time but also helps prevent impulsive food choices that may not align with your nutritional goals.

Regularly reviewing and adjusting your plan is also crucial for long-term success. As you progress on your nutritional journey, you may discover new foods or strategies that work better for you. Stay open-minded and be willing to adapt your plan accordingly. Remember, nutrition is not a one-size-fits-all approach, and what works for one person may not work for another.

Lastly, it is important to practice self-compassion and forgiveness throughout your journey towards sustaining optimal nutrition. There may be times when you deviate from your plan or make less healthy choices. Instead of dwelling on these setbacks, focus on the progress you have made and use them as learning opportunities. Remember that achieving optimal nutrition is a lifelong process, and it's okay to have occasional indulgences or setbacks as long as they are balanced with overall healthy habits.

By implementing these strategies and developing a long-term plan for sustaining optimal nutrition, you can enjoy the benefits of improved health and well-being for years to come.

11.3 Resources for Further Learning and Support

As you continue your journey towards optimal nutrition, it is essential to have access to resources that can provide further learning and support. Fortunately, there are numerous sources available that can help deepen your understanding of nutrition and offer guidance along the way.

One valuable resource is reputable websites dedicated to providing evidence-based information on nutrition. Websites such as the Academy of Nutrition and Dietetics (www.eatright.org) or the National Institutes of Health (www.nih.gov) offer a wealth of information on various aspects of nutrition, including dietary guidelines, nutrient databases, and educational materials.

Books written by experts in the field of nutrition can also provide valuable insights into achieving optimal nutrition. Look for books authored by registered dietitians or renowned researchers who specialize in nutrition. These books often delve deeper into specific topics related to nutrition and offer practical advice based on scientific evidence.

Podcasts focused on nutrition can be an excellent source of information while providing an engaging format for learning. Many podcasts feature interviews with experts in the field, discussing the latest research and trends in nutrition. Look for podcasts that align with your specific interests or goals, whether it's weight management, sports nutrition, or plant-based diets.

If you prefer a more interactive approach to learning, consider enrolling in online courses or workshops on nutrition. Many universities and organizations offer online programs that cover various aspects of nutrition, from basic concepts to advanced topics. These courses often provide a structured curriculum and allow you to interact with instructors and fellow learners.

Lastly, seeking guidance from a registered dietitian can be immensely beneficial in your journey towards optimal nutrition. Dietitians are trained professionals who can provide personalized advice based on your specific needs and goals. They can help you develop a customized meal plan, address any nutritional deficiencies or concerns, and offer ongoing support and accountability.

Remember that everyone's nutritional needs are unique, so it is essential to consult reliable sources and seek professional guidance when necessary. By utilizing these resources for further learning and support, you can continue expanding your knowledge of nutrition and receive the assistance needed to sustain optimal nutrition in the long term.

In conclusion, this comprehensive guide has provided valuable insights into achieving optimal nutrition. By recapping key concepts such as balanced diets, macronutrients, micronutrients, meal planning, portion control, and hydration, we have equipped you with the knowledge necessary to make informed choices about your diet. Additionally, by exploring strategies for sustaining optimal nutrition in the long term and providing resources for further learning and support, we have set you up for continued success on your nutritional journey. Remember that achieving optimal nutrition is a lifelong process that requires dedication and consistency. So take what you have learned from this guide and start making positive changes towards better health today!

Summary

"How to Get Enough Nutrition" is a comprehensive guide that aims to help individuals improve their diet and ensure they are getting all the necessary nutrients for optimal health. The book covers a wide range of topics related to nutrition, providing practical tips and advice for achieving a balanced diet.

The book begins by emphasizing the nutrition in daily life and the benefits it can bring to overall well-being. It highlights the struggles many people face in getting enough nutrition and offers solutions to optimize meals and ensure essential nutrients are included.

Extensive research has been conducted to provide accurate and up-to-date information on nutrition. Data, statistics, and trends have been analyzed to ensure the content is reliable. Keyword research has also been done to make the book more visible to readers.

To stand out from existing books on nutrition, the authors have studied their key features, strengths, and weaknesses. This allows them to offer unique insights into getting enough nutrition.

Expert guidance has been sought from professionals in the field of nutrition. Their expertise has helped determine the topics that should be addressed in the book and the most effective approaches for reaching the target audience.

The main topics covered in this book include understanding macronutrients and micronutrients, meal planning, portion control, and achieving a balanced diet. The authors provide practical tips on how to incorporate these concepts into daily life.

The tone of the book is informative and educational, presenting complex concepts in a clear and accessible manner. Natural language processing techniques have been used to identify keywords that will resonate with the target audience.

Overall, "How to Get Enough Nutrition" is a valuable resource for individuals looking to improve their diet and overall health. With its comprehensive coverage of various topics related to nutrition and its evidence-based approach backed by research findings and expert insights, this book provides readers with practical strategies for achieving optimal nutrition.

www.ingramcontent.com/pod-product-compliance
Lightning Source LLC
Chambersburg PA
CBHW070759260726
48660CB00005B/1690